GW00692105

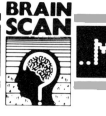

BRAIN
SCAN

Peter G. Elliott

MRCGP

Springer-Verlag
London Berlin Heidelberg New York
Paris Tokyo Hong Kong

Peter G. Elliott, BSc, Mb ChB, DRCOG, MRCGP
Bryn Awelon, The Castle, Denbigh, Clwyd LL16 3NB, Wales, UK

Publisher's note: the "Brainscan" logo is reproduced by courtesy of The Editor,
Geriatric Medicine, Modern Medicine GB Ltd.

ISBN 3-540-19563-7 Springer-Verlag Berlin Heidelberg New York
ISBN 0-387-19563-7 Springer-Verlag New York Berlin Heidelberg

British Library Cataloguing in Publication Data
Elliott, Peter G. *1947–*
　MRCGP, – Springer-Verlag *1989*
　1. General practice
　I. Title　II. Series
　362.1'72
　ISBN 3-540-19563-7

Library of Congress Cataloging-in-Publication Data
Elliott, Peter G., 1947–
　MRCGP.
　(Brainscan MCQ's)
　Bibliography: p.
　1. Internal medicine—Examinations, questions, etc.　I. Title.　II. Series.
RC58.E44　1989　616'.0076　　　　　　　　　　　　　　89-11498
ISBN 0-387-19563-7

Filmset by Macmillan India Ltd., Bangalore 25
Printed by The Bath Press, Bath, Avon
2128/3916-543210 (Printed on acid-free paper)

Preface

This book contains 300 multiple choice questions and is equivalent to five full MRCGP examinations. However, the layout is not as five examinations, but in the 15 subjects which have been chosen as relevant to general practice by the MCQ group of the Royal College of General Practitioners Examiners. I hope that using this format of individual sections will enable the book to have a wider use than just as a crammer for the exam: it should also serve as an aid to trainers and course organisers in assessing trainees during their vocational training. The questions themselves are in the usual multiple choice style with a stem followed by five responses, which can be answered true, false or don't know. The usual scoring method for examinations is $+1$ for a true, -1 for a false and 0 for a don't know.

In keeping with the current thinking of the College MCQ group, the stems have been kept as short as possible and an attempt has been made to adhere to standard nomenclature. For the purposes of this book the most common words used can be defined as follows:

Characteristic	– absence of this feature would cast doubt on the diagnosis
Typical	– would be expected but not as absolute a characteristic
Recognised	– a fact or an association that one would expect to be referred to in most standard textbooks or review articles on the subject
Has been shown	– a fact that has been reported so often as to gain the accolade of truth!
Majority	– greater than 50%

Wherever possible I have tried to avoid absolute figures, so generally it will be greater or less than a certain number that is asked for in a question, not the precise statistic. Sometimes in multiple choice questions the wording becomes a little contrived. I hope that the reader will bear with me in any such cases, which derive from the attempt to eliminate ambiguities that may arise when answering the questions.

I would like to thank the other members of the Royal College MCQ group for their help with some of the questions; they are Dr. Paul

Lewis, Dr. Julian Turner, Dr. Joe Butt, Dr. Stephen Murray and Dr. Jim McKellican. Finally I would like to thank Mrs. Karen Rizzi for typing the manuscript so excellently.

Denbigh   Peter Elliott

The MRCGP Examination

The MRCGP examination is held twice yearly and at present (1989) about 2000 candidates sit it each year.

It consists of five parts, each of which has an equal weighting; therefore the multiple choice section is worth 20% of the total marks. The other written sections are an MEQ and an essay type of question known as the PTQ. Candidates who obtain sufficient marks on the three written sections of the paper are invited to either Edinburgh or London to sit two separate oral examinations. The first of these is based on a log diary which the candidate presents, while the second is a more free-ranging viva involving topics chosen by the pair of examiners conducting the oral examination.

The MCQ has always been considered part of the examination which deals best with factual knowledge; other parts deal with patient management and attributes. Recent opinion within the College has considered that there ought to be a pass mark for the MCQ below which the candidate is not allowed to sit the rest of the examination. Therefore, it is prudent for candidates sitting the MRCGP to obtain as much practice as possible at multiple choice questions.

Below is a list of the 15 subjects chosen as relevant by the College MCQ group, together with the number of questions pertaining to them in an examination and in this book.

Topic	Exam	Book
General medicine	10	50
Psychiatry	6	30
Obstetrics and gynaecology	6	30
Therapeutics	6	30
Paediatrics	5	25
Surgery	3	15
ENT	2	10
Dermatology	4	20
Ophthalmology	3	15
Legal/ethical	2	10
Epidemiology/research	2	10

Topic	Exam	Book
Practice organisation	4	20
Care of the elderly	2	10
Physical medicine/trauma	3	15
Infectious disease	2	10
	60	300

Contents

1. General Medicine

Q.1.1 **When estimating plasma lipids:**

    a. A test performed within 3 weeks of a myocardial infarction will be an accurate basis for treatment

    b. HDL cholesterol varies with age

    c. Lipids are typically raised in patients receiving long-term dialysis

    d. Excessive alcohol intake raises lipid levels

    e. Failure to decrease cholesterol levels despite strict adherence to an adequate diet suggests a genetic cause

Q.1.2 **The following conditions have been shown to cause constipation:**

    a. Early pregnancy

    b. Hyperkalaemia

    c. Depression

    d. Hyperthyroidism

    e. Hypercalcaemia

Q.1.3 **The following conditions typically cause an eosinophilia in the peripheral blood film:**

    a. Dermatitis herpetiformis

    b. Atopic eczema

    c. Polyarteritis nodosa

    d. Burns

    e. Toxoplasmosis

Q.1.4 **Typical features of Addisonian pernicious anaemia include:**

    a. Intermittent glossitis

    b. Black hair

    c. Increased incidence of carcinoma of the stomach

    d. Mental changes

    e. Pyrexia

For answers see over

Answers

A.1.1 a. F—A test is only accurate within 24 hours of an attack or more than 3 months after one.
      b. F—It is LDL that varies with age, not HDL.
      c. T
      d. T
      e. T—A diet of less than 30% fat and only 10% saturated fat which fails to return levels to normal suggests familial hyperlipidaemia.

A.1.2 a. T
      b. F—Hypokalaemia does.
      c. T
      d. F—But myxoedema does.
      e. T

A.1.3 a. T
      b. T
      c. T
      d. F—They cause a leucocytosis.
      e. F—It causes a lymphocytosis.

A.1.4 a. T
      b. F—The hair is usually fair with premature greying.
      c. T
      d. T—Demyelination can give rise to peripheral and central nervous involvement.
      e. T—The pyrexia is usually mild.

Q.1.5 **Gingival swelling has been shown to be caused by:**

a. Combined oral contraceptives
b. Scurvy
c. Iron deficiency
d. Lichen planus
e. Phenytoin

Q.1.6 **Gynaecomastia has been shown to occur in:**

a. Renal failure treated by dialysis
b. Cirrhosis
c. Spironolactone therapy
d. "Normal" male puberty
e. Klinefelter's syndrome

Q.1.7 **The following are typical features of ulcerative colitis:**

a. An abdominal mass
b. Malabsorption
c. Bloody diarrhoea
d. A raised ESR
e. An increased frequency in Western Society

Q.1.8 **Farmer's lung (extrinsic allergic alveolitis):**

a. Presentation is typically with a flu-like illness
b. A normal chest X-ray excludes the diagnosis
c. The prevalence is increased in cigarette smokers
d. The patient is liable to benefit from an Industrial Injuries claim.
e. Clubbing of the fingers typically results from chronic exposure.

Q.1.9 **The following features support a diagnosis of systemic lupus erythematosus:**

a. Positive serological tests for syphilis
b. Preceding history of drug allergies
c. Alopecia
d. Photosensitivity of the skin
e. Thrombocytopenia

For answers see over

Answers

A.1.5 a. T
　　　　b. T
　　　　c. F—Iron deficiency causes stomatitis.
　　　　d. F—Lichen planus causes stomatitis.
　　　　e. T

A.1.6 a. T
　　　　b. T
　　　　c. T
　　　　d. T
　　　　e. T

A.1.7 a. F—This is typically a feature of Crohn's disease.
　　　　b. F—As there is no small bowel involvement.
　　　　c. T—It is less common in Crohn's disease.
　　　　d. T—The ESR is usually very high in the acute attack.
　　　　e. T—There is also an increasing prevalence in those societies developing Western diets, e.g. Japan.

A.1.8 a. T—The commonest presentation.
　　　　b. F—Typical changes resolve quickly after the exposure to the allergen ceases.
　　　　c. F—Because the immune response of smokers is depressed.
　　　　d. T
　　　　e. F

A.1.9 a. T—SLE is commonest cause of a false-positive.
　　　　b. T
　　　　c. T
　　　　d. T—Sunlight can exacerbate the joint pain and stiffness.
　　　　e. T

Q.1.10 Aortic stenosis:

a. Angina pectoris has been shown to be present in the absence of coexisting coronary artery disease
b. A normal chest X-ray excludes the diagnosis
c. A normal electrocardiograph excludes the diagnosis
d. It occurs most commonly in elderly females
e. Valve replacement is the treatment of choice

Q.1.11 Obesity:

a. Oral contraceptives cause an increase in energy expenditure
b. Body mass index is calculated by dividing the patient's weight in kilograms by the square of the height in metres
c. Smoking does not increase energy expenditure
d. 1300 kcal per day typically produces weight loss in the majority of adult men
e. 400 kcal is the recommended minimum daily requirement of a very low calorie diet

Q.1.12 The following are recognised causes of atrial fibrillation:

a. Anxiety
b. Hyperthyroidism
c. Ventricular septal defect
d. Alcohol abuse
e. Pulmonary embolism

Q.1.13 The following are recognised causes of Cheyne-Stokes breathing:

a. Head injury
b. Diabetic coma
c. Uraemia
d. Meningitis
e. Left ventricular failure

For answers see over

Answers

A.1.10 a. T—The angina resolves after valve replacement.
        b. F—Cardiac enlargement is unusual and indicates a degree of aortic incompetence.
        c. F—A normal ECG can occur in severe stenosis.
        d. F—It is most common in elderly males.
        e. T—Due to the risk of sudden death medical treatment of symptoms is unsatisfactory.

A.1.11 a. F—The Pill inhibits ovulation; therefore the rise in body temperature (and basal metabolic rate) does not occur.
        b. T—Remember that the formula does not work if calculated in imperial measures.
        c. F—One cigarette accounts for 9 kcal of energy expenditure.
        d. T—But everybody will lose weight on an 800 kcal diet.
        e. T—But 500 kcal is recommended for all men and women over 5 ft 8 in.

A.1.12 a. F—Anxiety causes sinus tachycardia.
        b. T—It also causes sinus tachycardia.
        c. F—But atrial septal defect is a cause.
        d. T
        e. T

A.1.13 a. T—Due to brain stem compression.
        b. F—Diabetic coma causes Kussmaul respiration.
        c. T—It is due to the metabolic upset.
        d. T—It is due to brain stem irritation.
        e. T

Q.1.14 **The risk of malignancy has been shown to be increased in association with:**

    a. Crohn's disease
    b. Familial polyposis coli
    c. Pernicious anaemia
    d. Coal dust exposure
    e. Ankylosing spondylitis

Q.1.15 **Trigeminal neuralgia:**

    a. The pain typically lasts for more than 5 min
    b. It has been shown to be associated with multiple sclerosis
    c. The pain is typically bilateral
    d. The majority of cases have a recognisable stimulus
    e. Removal of retained dental roots has been shown to be curative in some cases

Q.1.16 **In cases of Guillain-Barré syndrome:**

    a. the course is typically slowly progressive
    b. reflexes are typically enhanced
    c. facial and cranial nerves are typically spared
    d. hearing loss is typical
    e. the majority of patients have an antecedent infection

Q.1.17 **Sarcoidosis:**

    a. When it is associated with bilateral hilar lymphadenopathy the prognosis is poor in the absence of treatment
    b. There is an association with hypercalcaemia
    c. Peak flow rates are characteristically reduced in pulmonary sarcoid
    d. Anterior uveitis is a typical feature
    e. Finger clubbing is a typical feature of the pulmonary disease

For answers see over

Answers

A.1.14 a. T
        b. T
        c. T—The incidence of carcinoma of the stomach is increased.
        d. F
        e. F—But patients who have received radiotherapy to the spine have an increased incidence of leukaemias.

A.1.15 a. F—The pain is usually fleeting.
        b. T—It is associated with multiple sclerosis in ca. 3% of cases.
        c. F—It is invariably unilateral.
        d. T—Usually eating, talking, washing or shaving.
        e. T—It is important to exclude a dental cause.

A.1.16 a. F—It is rapidly progressive.
        b. F—They are absent.
        c. F—Facial weakness is common.
        d. F—Hearing loss is unknown.
        e. T—66% have a definite history of infection within the 3 months preceding infection.

A.1.17 a. F—The prognosis is good.
        b. T—10%–20% of patients.
        c. F—Severe radiographic changes may be associated with normal pulmonary function tests.
        d. T—Eyes should be examined under the slit lamp as they may be asymptomatic.
        e. F—It is uncommon except in advanced cases of pulmonary fibrosis.

Q.1.18   Huntington's disease:

a. Inheritance is autosomal recessive
b. The mean age of onset is 40 years
c. New mutations account for the majority of cases
d. Paternal transmission to children typically leads to an early onset of the disease
e. CT scanning typically shows changes in the brain

Q.1.19   Subacute bacterial endocarditis is associated with:

a. Recent sigmoidoscopy
b. Café-au-lait patches on the skin
c. Patent ductus arteriosus
d. Petechiae on the skin
e. Haematuria on dipstick testing of the urine

Q.1.20   Mitral valve prolapse

a. is associated with mitral stenosis
b. is associated with coronary heart disease
c. is a risk factor for subacute bacterial endocarditis
d. is present in the majority of patients with Marfan's syndrome
e. typically produces a systolic click

Q.1.21   Gilbert's syndrome:

a. The serum alkaline phosphatase concentration is typically raised above normal
b. Characteristically the level of icterus is variable
c. The liver typically shows no histological abnormality
d. The urine typically shows excess urobilinogen
e. There is typically a familial distribution

Q.1.22   Splenomegaly is a recognised feature of:

a. Thyrotoxicosis
b. Carcinoma of the pancreas
c. Rheumatoid arthritis
d. Schistosomiasis
e. Gluten enteropathy

For answers see over

Answers

A.1.18   a. F—Inheritance is autosomal dominant; therefore 50% of offspring will be affected.
          b. T
          c. F—New mutations are rare.
          d. T
          e. T—Atrophy of the caudate nucleus.

A.1.19   a. F—Antibiotic cover is not usual for this procedure.
          b. F—Such patches are associated with neurofibromatosis.
          c. T
          d. T
          e. T

A.1.20   a. F
          b. T
          c. T
          d. T
          e. T

A.1.21   a. F—The only abnormality is a raised bilirubin level.
          b. T
          c. T
          d. F
          e. T—It is the commonest form of familial non-haemolytic hyperbilirubinaemia, affecting 2%-5% of the population.

A.1.22   a. T—5% of those with Graves' disease show splenomegaly.
          b. T—Secondary to splenic vein thrombosis.
          c. T—Felty's syndrome.
          d. T—The spleen is usually massive.
          e. F—There is usually splenic atrophy.

Q.1.23 **Oat cell carcinoma of the bronchus**

   a. is typically radiosensitive
   b. occurs with equal frequency in smokers and non-smokers
   c. has a 5-year survival greater than 20%
   d. has been shown to cause hyponatraemia
   e. is the commonest cause of ectopic parathormone secretion

Q.1.24 **Migrainous neuralgia (cluster headache):**

   a. It is more common in men than women
   b. A family history is typical
   c. The pain is characteristically bilateral
   d. Nausea has been shown to be more common than with classical migraine
   e. Alcohol typically provokes an attack of pain

Q.1.25 **Parkinson's disease:**

   a. An association with dysphagia has been shown
   b. The majority of patients are above their optimal weight
   c. Tremor is typically unilateral in the early stages
   d. Constipation is characteristic
   e. There is an association with accelerated mental retardation

Q.1.26 **The following conditions have been shown to be risk factors for cerebral infarction:**

   a. Atrial fibrillation
   b. Diabetes mellitus
   c. Oral contraceptive therapy
   d. Plasma fibrinogen above normal levels
   e. Ischaemic heart disease

For answers see over

Answers

A.1.23 a. F—It is very radioresistant.
          b. F—Adenocarcinoma is not cigarette dependent.
          c. F—The 5-year survival rate is less than 5%.
          d. T—Due to inappropriate secretion of antidiuretic hormone.
          e. T

A.1.24 a. T—Unlike classical migraine, which is more common in women.
          b. F
          c. F—It is strictly unilateral.
          d. F—It is less common.
          e. T

A.1.25 a. T—Due to stasis and irregular contractions of the epiglottis.
          b. F—75% are below the mean weight for their height and age.
          c. T—So is the rigidity.
          d. T—Megacolon may occur.
          e. T—Depression is also typical.

A.1.26 a. T
          b. T
          c. T
          d. T
          e. T

Q.1.27 **Bell's palsy:**
a. An association with diabetes mellitus has been shown
b. It is a recognised complication of severe hypertension
c. Numbness of the affected side of the face excludes the diagnosis
d. The majority of patients make a complete recovery without treatment
e. Corticosteroids have been shown to be effective in decreasing the severity of symptoms

Q.1.28 **Occupational asthma has been shown to be caused by:**
a. Asbestos
b. Nickel
c. Epoxy resins
d. Biological enzymes
e. Mahogany

Q.1.29 **In differentiating between epilepsy and syncope, a diagnosis of epilepsy would be supported by:**
a. Pallor
b. Bradycardia
c. Sweating
d. Nocturnal attacks
e. Faecal incontinence

Q.1.30 **Proteinuria in the absence of renal disease has been shown to occur in:**
a. Joggers
b. Febrile upper respiratory tract infection
c. Congestive cardiac failure
d. Diabetes mellitus
e. Hypertension

For answers see over

Answers

A.1.27   a. T
b. T
c. F—Such numbness is attributed to trigeminal nerve involvement.
d. T
e. T—Treatment is usually with an initial dose of 80 mg/day, decreasing over 10 days.

A.1.28   a. F
b. T—In welders.
c. T—In adhesive manufacturing.
d. T—In the pharmaceutical industry.
e. T—In carpenters.

A.1.29   a. F
b. F
c. F
d. F
e. T—Faecal incontinence is even more diagnostic of epilepsy than urinary incontinence.

A.1.30   a. T—Haematuria may also occur after violent exertion.
b. T—In approximately 5% of cases.
c. T—It resolves after treatment of the failure.
d. F
e. F

Q.1.31 Relative polycythaemia:

a. There is an association with decreased cerebral blood flow
b. An association with diuretic therapy has been shown
c. The majority of cases occur in cigarette smokers
d. The red cell mass is charateristically elevated above normal
e. A genetic component has been demonstrated

Q.1.32 In differentiating between pulmonary embolism and myocardial infarction the following would support the latter diagnosis:

a. Cyanosis
b. Pain aggravated by inspiration
c. Cough
d. Pleural rub
e. Onset of atrial fibrillation

Q.1.33 Spontaneous pneumothorax

a. is more common in women than in men
b. typically occurs in the elderly
c. recurs in the majority of patients
d. is associated with chronic obstructive airways disease
e. has been shown to be more common at the time of menstruation

Q.1.34 Obesity has been shown to be associated with:

a. Amenorrhoea
b. Impairment of glucose tolerance
c. Decreased thyroxine levels
d. Elevated cortisol levels
e. Cardiac hypertrophy

For answers see over

Answers

A.1.31 a. T—And therefore the risk of cerebral infarction is increased.

          b. T—There is an association with anything which dehydrates the patient, e.g. alcohol.

          c. T

          d. F—Such elevation suggests another cause for the polycythaemia.

          e. T—But it is ill-defined.

A.1.32 a. F

          b. F

          c. F

          d. F

          e. T

A.1.33 a. F—The male-female ratio is 5:1.

          b. F—It typically occurs in young adults.

          c. F—It recurs in one-third if untreated.

          d. T—It often accounts for a sudden worsening of asthma or emphysema.

          e. T—The association is usually with a left-sided pneumothorax.

A.1.34 a. T

          b. T—Such impairment is usually related to the duration of obesity.

          c. F

          d. F

          e. T—The hypertrophy usually reverses on loss of weight.

Q.1.35 Paracetamol poisoning:

    a. In an adult a dose of 25 g is typically fatal without treatment

    b. Children are less tolerant than adults of paracetamol over-dosage

    c. Oral methionine is only effective if given within 10 h of ingestion

    d. Most of the drug is excreted unchanged in the urine

    e. Signs of hepatic damage typically develop within 2–3 days

Q.1.36 The following have been shown to cause a decrease in plasma calcium:

    a. Osteogenesis imperfecta

    b. Osteoporosis

    c. Osteomalacia

    d. Renal failure

    e. Rickets

Q.1.37 Primary biliary cirrhosis

    a. typically presents with pruritus

    b. has been shown to be associated with Hashimoto's thyroiditis

    c. typically causes finger clubbing

    d. is associated with dermatomyosites

    e. is commoner in men than women

Q.1.38 Gluten is found in:

    a. Oats

    b. Rye

    c. Wheat

    d. Barley

    e. Rice

For answers see over

Answers

A.1.35 a. T—15 g is likely to cause severe liver damage.
      b. F—They are more tolerant.
      c. T
      d. F
      e. T

A.1.36 a. F—The problem is collagen metabolism.
      b. F—Calcium levels are normal.
      c. T
      d. T
      e. T

A.1.37 a. T—In 70% of patients.
      b. T—Both are auto-immune connective tissue disorders.
      c. T
      d. T—Dermatomyositis is also an auto-immune connective tissue disorder.
      e. F—90% of cases occur in women.

A.1.38 a. T
      b. T
      c. T
      d. T
      e. T

Q.1.39 It has been shown that the prognosis following myocardial infarction is improved by:

a. Cessation of cigarette smoking
b. Weight reduction
c. Correction of hyperlipidaemia
d. Physical exercise
e. Control of blood pressure

Q.1.40 Mesothelioma

a. has been shown to be more prevalent after exposure to blue asbestos rather than white asbestos
b. is more common in asbestos workers who smoke
c. typically presents with a pleural effusion
d. typically responds to chemotherapy
e. has a prognosis which is uninfluenced by treatment

Q.1.41 Recognised features of gluten-sensitive enteropathy are:

a. Spontaneous remission of symptoms
b. An increased risk of carcinoma
c. Excessive bruising
d. Polyarthralgia
e. Aphthous ulceration

Q.1.42 Crohn's disease:

a. Viral infection has been shown to be the cause
b. Typically the whole gastrointestinal tract apart from the stomach is affected
c. The majority of patients will require surgery at some stage in the course of their disease
d. It has been shown to cause vitamin B_{12} deficiency
e. A high fibre diet is indicated in the presence of strictures

For answers see over

Answers

A.1.39 a. T
          b. F
          c. F
          d. F
          e. F

A.1.40 a. T
          b. F—But they are more likely to develop cancer of the lung.
          c. T—And chest pain and dyspnoea.
          d. F
          e. T—Prognosis is usually months only.

A.1.41 a. T—Often for long periods.
          b. T—There is an increased incidence not just of carcinoma of the small bowel but of carcinoma generally.
          c. T—Due to vitamin K deficiency.
          d. F
          e. T

A.1.42 a. F
          b. F—But the whole gastrointestinal tract apart from the stomach *can* be affected.
          c. T—Approximately 75% do so.
          d. T—Due to decreased absorption from an affected terminal ileum.
          e. F—In the presence of strictures a high fibre diet can reduce obstruction. Therefore a low fibre diet is indicated.

Q.1.43   Hodgkin's disease:

    a. The incidence is higher in those who have undergone tonsillectomy
    b. It is commoner in women than in men
    c. Constitutional symptoms are associated with a worse prognosis
    d. Cervical lymphadenopathy is classically painful
    e. CT scanning has replaced staging laparotomy

Q.1.44   Multiple myeloma may present with:

    a. Bone pain
    b. Renal failure
    c. Hypercalcaemia
    d. Bleeding
    c. Fever

Q.1.45   Carotid sinus massage has been shown to be of value in the treatment of:

    a. Atrial fibrillation
    b. Atrial flutter
    c. Paroxysmal ventricular tachycardia
    d. Sinus bradycardia
    e. Tachycardia associated with Wolff-Parkinson-White syndrome

Q.1.46   The following have been shown to be risk factors for deep venous thrombosis:

    a. Connective tissue disease
    b. Cigarette smoking
    c. Obesity
    d. Heart failure
    e. Malignant disease

For answers see over

Answers

A.1.43 a. T
b. F—The male-female ratio is 3:2.
c. T—Except pruritus.
d. F—It is painless.
e. F—CT is unable to detect micro-involvement of the liver or spleen.

A.1.44 a. T—70%.
b. T—10%.
c. T—20%.
d. T—10%.
e. T—15%.

A.1.45 a. T
b. T
c. T
d. F
e. F

A.1.46 a. T
b. F—It may be a negative risk factor.
c. T
d. T
e. T

Q.1.47 Myalgic encephalomyelitis:

    a. Lack of demonstrable exercise-induced muscle fatigue excludes the diagnosis
    b. Loss of short-term memory is typical
    c. Night sweats are a typical finding
    d. The majority of patients show Coxsackie IgM antibodies
    e. The ESR is characteristically elevated above normal values

Q.1.48 The following would be compatible with a diagnosis of pulmonary oedema due to left ventricular failure:

    a. Sinus tachycardia
    b. Normal blood pressure
    c. Jugular venous pressure that is not elevated
    d. Pleural effusion
    e. A wheezy chest

Q.1.49 Diabetes mellitus:

    a. A random blood glucose of 7 mmol/l excludes the diagnosis
    b. A glucose tolerance test is mandatory in all suspected diabetics
    c. Ideally carbohydrate should contribute more than 50% of the diet
    d. Glycosylated haemoglobin provides a measure of control over the preceding 6 months
    e. One gram of fat provides more than twice as much energy as one gram of carbohydrate

Q.1.50 The following factors increase the risk of death during admission to hospital with a myocardial infarction:

    a. Inferior rather than anterior infarction pattern on the ECG
    b. Age over 65 years rather than under 65 years
    c. A persistent low blood pressure
    d. Tachycardia
    e. A previous myocardial infarction

For answers see over

Answers

A.1.47 a. T—This must be present before the diagnosis can be made.
  b. T—This improves with rest.
  c. T—Along with other symptoms of autonomic dysfunction.
  d. F—Only 10%-20% do so.
  e. F—It is usually normal.

A.1.48 a. T
  b. T—Blood pressure may be normal, elevated or low.
  c. F—It is always elevated in pulmonary oedema due to solely left ventricular failure.
  d. T
  e. T—Usually accompanied by fine crackles at the lung bases.

A.1.49 a. T—The accepted upper level of normal is 8 mmol/l; above 11 mmol/l is virtually diagnostic.
  b. F—It is rarely necessary.
  c. T—Usually 50%-60%, but preferably complex carbohydrate.
  d. F—It does so for 2–3 months.
  e. T

A.1.50 a. F—The reverse is true.
  b. T—30% vs 15%.
  c. T
  d. F—Tachycardia often occurs due to pain and anxiety.
  e. T

2. *Psychiatry*

Q.2.1   Bulimia nervosa

    a. typically involves an obsessional personality
    b. typically develops earlier than anorexia nervosa
    c. has a better outome than anorexia nervosa
    d. is associated with laxative abuse
    e. is typically accompanied by excessive dental caries

Q.2.2   Puerperal psychosis:

    a. Onset is typically within 10 days of delivery
    b. The majority of women have a recurrence of the illness in subsequent pregnancies
    c. Rejection of the baby is characteristic
    d. Affective features are typical
    e. There is typically a previous psychiatric history

Q.2.3   The following have been shown to be good prognostic indicators in schizophrenia:

    a. Gradual onset of symptoms
    b. Known precipitating cause
    c. Flattening of affect
    d. Family history of schizophrenia
    e. Prominent affective symptoms

Q.2.4   The following factors typically indicate that an attempted suicide was of serious intent:

    a. A suicide note
    b. Informing others of the intention before the attempt
    c. Making a will before the attempt
    d. Admitting suicidal intent
    e. Hoarding tablets for the attempt

For answers see over

Answers

A.2.1 a. T—And a higher socio-economic group.
        b. F—Mean onset is at 17–18 years as opposed to 13–14 years for anorexia.
        c. T—50% maintain remission.
        d. T
        e. T—Due to the effect of excessive sweet foods and vomiting.

A.2.2 a. T
        b. F—The rate of recurrence is approximately 20%.
        c. F—It is best to admit both mother and baby if possible.
        d. T—So typical that puerperal psychosis is considered a variant of manic-depressive illness by many psychiatrists.
        e. F

A.2.3 a. F—An acute onset usually has a better outlook.
        b. T
        c. F
        d. F
        e. T

A.2.4 a. T
        b. T
        c. T
        d. T
        e. T

Q.2.5 First rank symptoms of schizophrenia include:

a. Thought insertion
b. Confabulation
c. Flattening of affect
d. Poverty of speech
e. Thought broadcasting

Q.2.6 The following have been shown to be associated with hysterical seizures:

a. Tongue biting
b. Immature personality
c. Normal flexor plantar response
d. Abnormal pupil response
e. A pre-existing history of established epilepsy

Q.2.7 Typical features of depressive illness include:

a. Flights of ideas
b. Anxiety
c. Impairment of recent memory
d. Difficulty in concentration
e. Spontaneous recovery

Q.2.8 Obsessional thoughts

a. are typically unpleasant
b. are associated with severe depressive illness
c. have been shown to improve with clomipramine therapy
d. typically respond to psychotherapy
e. resolve spontaneously in the majority of patients

Q.2.9 The following are typical features of Korsakoff's syndrome:

a. Impairment of recent memory
b. Chronic alcoholism
c. Confabulation
d. Association with peripheral neuritis
e. Association with ophthalmoplegia

For answers see over

Answers

A.2.5 a. T—Experiencing thoughts being put into one's mind.
　　　b. F—This is typical of Korsakoff's psychosis.
　　　c. F—This is not a first rank symptom.
　　　d. F—Again, this is not a first rank symptom.
　　　e. T—Experiencing one's thoughts being known to other people.

A.2.6 a. T—And incontinence may occur.
　　　b. T—There will often have been previous attention-seeking behaviour.
　　　c. T
　　　d. F
　　　e. T

A.2.7 a. F—Suggests hypomania.
　　　b. T
　　　c. F—Suggests associated dementia.
　　　d. T
　　　e. T

A.2.8 a. F—But they may be aggressive, sexual or obscene.
　　　b. T—Or with schizophrenia.
　　　c. T—Clomipramine is the tricyclic antidepressant of choice.
　　　d. F—They are usually resistant.
　　　e. F—The majority develop a chronic obsessive-compulsive neurosis.

A.2.9 a. T
　　　b. T
　　　c. T—Invention of stories to fill in memory gaps.
　　　d. T
　　　e. T

Q.2.10 A normal grief reaction would be indicated by:

a. Inability to express any emotion in the week following death of a spouse
b. Suicidal thoughts 4 weeks after bereavement
c. Prolonged absence from work 3 months after bereavement
d. A feeling that the dead person is still present 1 month after their death
e. Insomnia 6 months after the funeral

Q.2.11 The following are typical feature of a manic disorder:

a. Increased libido
b. Increased appetite
c. Expansive ideas
d. Clouding of consciousness
e. Thought broadcasting

Q.2.12 Hypochondriasis:

a. There is a characteristic association with an obsessional personality
b. Schizophrenia has been shown to present in this way
c. There is an association with depressive illness
d. There is typically a response to treatment with monoamine oxidase inhibitors
e. Studies have shown that psychogenic pain is over-diagnosed

Q.2.13 Senile dementia

a. typically has an abrupt onset
b. typically produces a fluctuating level of consciousness
c. has been shown to occur more frequently in first-degree relatives of those affected
d. typically involves outbursts of tears and anger
e. is typically aggravated by physical illness, if the dementia is mild

For answers see over

Answers

A.2.10 a. T—This stage may last up to 2 weeks.
      b. T—Such thoughts are associated with guilt and a feeling of responsibility for the death.
      c. F—This indicates social isolation; usually no more than 2 weeks are taken off work.
      d. T—This feeling is often still present after 6 months.
      e. T

A.2.11 a. T
      b. T
      c. T
      d. F—Indicates an organic brain disorder.
      e. F—First rank symptom of schizophrenia.

A.2.12 a. F—Any personality type is vulnerable.
      b. T
      c. T—Especially if the hypochondriacal symptoms are severe.
      d. F—Drug therapy is only of use in treating associated psychiatric illness.
      e. T

A.2.13 a. F—It is more likely to be a confusional state.
      b. F—Head injury with or without a subdural haematoma would be more likely to do this.
      c. T—There is a slightly increased risk in first-degree relatives.
      d. F—Such outbursts are typical of multi-infarct dementia.
      e. T—Such aggravation is typically reversed on dealing with the physical problem.

Q.2.14 The following features are typical of delirium tremens:

a. Prolonged insomnia
b. Disorientation in time and place
c. Misinterpretation of sensory stimuli
d. Course lasting 3 or 4 days
e. The patient is able to recall the delirious period after it is over

Q.2.15 Electroconvulsive therapy:

a. It is contra-indicated in the elderly
b. Unilateral ECT has less pronounced side-effects than bipolar treatment
c. Muscle relaxants are given prior to treatment
d. Short-term memory loss has been shown to occur after treatment
e. It can be given against the patient's wishes under Section 2 of the Mental Health Act

Q.2.16 Depression in the elderly:

a. The depression is typically reactive
b. There is a greater risk of suicide than among younger patients
c. Weight loss is typical
d. There is a typical history of depression in earlier life
e. Social isolation is a typical precipitating cause

Q.2.17 Agoraphobia:

a. Women are more commonly affected than men
b. The mean age of onset is 30–40 years
c. There is a typical history of neurotic disorder in childhood
d. The majority of sufferers experience depersonalization
e. Attacks have been shown to be less likely in places where there are a lot of people.

For answers see over

Answers

A.2.14 a. T
       b. T
       c. T—There are also vivid hallucinations in all modalities.
       d. T
       e. F—The patient has little memory of the events.

A.2.15 a. F—It is only contra-indicated if the patient is confused following anaesthesia.
       b. T
       c. T
       d. T
       e. F—Usually under Section 3 and with a second opinion from the mental health commissioner.

A.2.16 a. F—Endogenous depression is common.
       b. T
       c. T—This may lead to a mistaken diagnosis of physical illness.
       d. F—Often the first attacks occur in 65–80 year olds.
       e. T

A.2.17 a. T
       b. F—Onset is usually between 15 and 30 years.
       c. T
       d. T—60%.
       e. F—They are more likely in crowded places and less likely in an open field.

Q.2.18   In cannabis abuse

   a. withdrawal symptoms are typical
   b. tolerance has been shown to occur
   c. cerebral atrophy has been demonstrated
   d. psychosis has been shown to occur
   e. teratogenicity has been demonstrated

Q.2.19   In the Mental Health Act of 1983

   a. dependence on alcohol is accepted as a reason for compulsory admission
   b. Section 2 requires the recommendation of a consultant psychiatrist
   c. Section 2 does not permit relatives to make an application for admission
   d. Section 3 allows admission for a maximum of 6 months
   e. Section 4 requires the recommendation of only one doctor

Q.2.20   Psychiatric manifestations of frontal lobe tumours include:

   a. Euphoria
   b. Sexual indiscretions
   c. Depression
   d. Memory loss
   e. Visual hallucinations

Q.2.21   Premature ejaculation

   a. is defined as the failure to satisfy the partner in 50% of coital attempts
   b. may be combatted by a reduction in the amount of foreplay
   c. may be combatted by thought distraction during intercourse
   d. may be alleviated by clomipramine
   e. may be alleviated by the squeeze technique

For answers see over

Answers

A.2.18 a. F
      b. F
      c. F—It has been reported but not substantiated.
      d. F—Not in the absence of other psychiatric illness.
      e. F—But abuse has not yet been proved safe.

A.2.19 a. F—Only if associated with another disorder.
      b. F—An approved doctor is suitable.
      c. F—They can, but it is usually done by a social worker.
      d. T
      e. T—But it only allows admission for 72 hours.

A.2.20 a. T—Over-talkativeness is common.
      b. T—A manifestation of disinhibition.
      c. F
      d. T—Usually the onset is slow.
      e. F

A.2.21 a. T—It is defined in this way by Masters and Johnson.
      b. F—This tends to make the situation worse.
      c. F—Again this tends to make things worse.
      d. T
      e. T—As described by Masters and Johnson.

Q.2.22 **The following factors have been shown to contribute to psychiatric problems after mutilating surgery:**

a. Pre-existing history of depressive illness
b. Physical complications post-operatively
c. Adverse experience in a close friend or relative
d. A feeling of lack of support
e. Increased age of the patient

Q.2.23 **In the mentally handicapped**

a. Alzheimer's disease has been shown to be more prevalent in the presence of Down's syndrome
b. benzodiazepines have been shown to cause disinhibition
c. schizophrenia is more common than in the general population
d. disturbed behaviour has been shown to be more common in the presence of depression
e. suicide has been shown to be rare when there are severe learning problems

Q.2.24 **The following psychiatric disorders have been shown to be more common in first-degree relatives:**

a. Alcoholism
b. Bipolar affective disorders
c. Schizophrenia
d. Alzheimer's disease
e. Psychotic depression

Q.2.25 **Following a suicide attempt the following have been shown to be prognostic indicators for the likelihood of a further attempt:**

a. Higher social class
b. Criminal record
c. Previous psychiatric treatment
d. Alcohol problems
e. Unemployment

For answers see over

Answers

A.2.22 a. T—Or of anxiety.
        b. T
        c. T
        d. T
        e. F—Psychiatric problems are not related to age.

A.2.23 a. T—This has been demonstrated by post-mortem examination.
        b. T—Insomnia is best treated by antihistamines.
        c. T
        d. T—Depression may be very difficult to diagnose.
        e. T—It is virtually unknown.

A.2.24 a. T—But it is difficult to seperate genetic from environmental factors.
        b. T—The risk is 5% vs 1% in the general population.
        c. T—There is a 40% risk in a monozygotic twin.
        d. T
        e. T

A.2.25 a. F—There is an association with lower social class membership.
        b. T
        c. T
        d. T
        e. T

Q.2.26 **The following drugs have been shown to cause hallucinations:**

a. Phenytoin
b. Digoxin
c. Penicillin
d. Pentazocine
e. Levadopa

Q.2.27 **Doctors have been shown to be more at risk from the following psychiatric disorders:**

a. Schizophrenia
b. Drug dependency
c. Alcoholism
d. Depression
e. Personality disorders

Q.2.28 **The following have been shown to be relevant to the development of behaviour disturbance in adolescence:**

a. Parental illness
b. Going to boarding school
c. Poverty
d. Divorce of parents
e. Being male rather than female

Q.2.29 **The following have been shown to be more common in women at the menopause:**

a. Hypomania
b. Schizophrenia
c. Alcohol-related problems
d. Insomnia
e. Poor concentration

For answers see over

Answers

A.2.26 a. F—It can cause delirium.
          b. T—It also causes delirium.
          c. F—But it can cause delirium.
          d. T
          e. T—It also causes behavioural changes and psychotic states.

A.2.27 a. F
          b. T
          c. T
          d. T
          e. F

A.2.28 a. T
          b. F
          c. T
          d. T
          e. T—It is much commoner in males.

A.2.29 a. F—But depressive illness is more common.
          b. F—It is more common in a younger age group.
          c. T
          d. T
          e. T

Q.2.30 **The following have been shown to be typical features of schizophrenia:**

    a. Flights of ideas
    b. Concrete thinking
    c. Hypochondriacal delusions
    d. Visual hallucinations
    e. Neologisms

For answers see over

Answers

A.2.30 a. F—They are more likely in manic depressive illness.
        b. T
        c. T
        d. F—They usually indicate an organic brain disorder.
        e. T

3. Obstetrics and Gynaecology

Questions

Q.3.1   Endometriosis

a. is the commonest cause of secondary dysmenorrhea
b. typically produces a colicky pain which starts on the first day of the period
c. produces symptoms the severity of which is proportional to the extensiveness of the disease
d. can sometimes be effectively treated by danazol
e. is associated with infertility

Q.3.2   Ectopic pregnancy:

a. The diagnosis is excluded by a history of regular menstruation
b. The left fallopian tube is affected significantly more often than the right
c. There is an association with a history of pelvic inflammatory disease
d. Vaginal examination should be performed prior to hospital referral
e. Typically there is an association with vaginal bleeding

Q.3.3   Post-coital contraception using the combined oral contraceptive

a. is available free of prescription charges
b. must be given within 24 hours of intercourse
c. has been shown to cause nausea and vomiting
d. is suitable as a long-term method of contraception if given on a regular basis at the time of ovulation
e. has a suitable alternative in the form of an intra-uterine device inserted 5 days after unprotected intercourse

Q.3.4   A raised serum alpha-fetoprotein level has been shown to be due to:

a. Multiple pregnancy
b. Missed abortion
c. Down's syndrome
d. Duchenne muscular dystrophy
e. Exomphalos

For answers see over

Answers

A.3.1. a. T
 b. F—The pain is continuous and starts before the period commences.
 c. F—Severe disease may produce few symptoms whereas mild disease can give severe symptoms.
 d. T—Danazol is the most popular treatment despite the cost.
 e. T—The two conditions occur together more commonly than can be explained by chance; the exact relationship has not been worked out.

A.3.2 a. F—It often occurs before the first "missed" period.
 b. The opposite is true allegedly owing to the proximity of the appendix.
 c. T—Adhesions and tubal damage.
 d. F—Such examination involves danger of rupture of the inflamed tube.
 e. T—But may occur in the absence of bleeding.

A.3.3 a. T—Sign a 1001.
 b. F—72 hours is the safe limit.
 c. T
 d. F—Too frequent repeats are not recommended because of the high oestrogenic component.
 e. T—IUDs were widely used before introduction of the drug method.

A.3.4 a. T
 b. T
 c. F—Chromosomal analysis of amniotic fluid is necessary for the diagnosis.
 d. T—A prenatal test has recently become available.
 e. T

Q.3.5 **Intra-uterine contraception devices are contra-indicated in the following:**

a. A history of pelvic inflammatory disease 5 years previously
b. Azathioprine therapy for Crohn's disease
c. A previous ectopic pregnancy
d. HIV positivity
e. Valvular heart disease

Q.3.6 **Premenstrual tension:**

a. Progestogen deficiency can be demonstrated in the majority of cases
b. Natural progestogen is available as an oral preparation
c. Natural progestogen in therapeutic doses acts as a contraceptive
d. Pyridoxine 50 mg daily has been shown to be significantly more effective than placebo in relieving symptoms
e. Occurrence is typically in the teenage and early twenty age groups

Q.3.7 **When considering drug therapy during pregnancy:**

a. Methyldopa is contra-indicated at all stages
b. Treatment with isotretinoin is a recognised indication for termination
c. Folic acid supplements should be given to patients taking phenytoin
d. Heparin has been shown to cause central nervous system damage in the foetus if given in the second and third trimesters
e. Thiazide diuretics have been shown to decrease placental perfusion

Q.3.8 **Pregnancy in teenagers under 16 years of age has**

a. the highest rate of maternal mortality of any age group
b. an increased stillbirth rate
c. an increased perinatal death rate
d. an increased neonatal death rate
e. an increased infant death rate

For answers see over

Answers

A.3.5 a. F—Only active pelvic inflammatory disease is an absolute contra-indication.
b. T—Immunosuppressive therapy is a contra-indication.
c. T—Use of IUDs is associated with an increased incidence of ectopic pregnancy.
d. T—IUDs affect the immune response
e. F—This is only a relative contra-indication.

A.3.6 a. F
b. F—It can only be given parenterally or as a pessary or suppository.
c. F
d. F
e. F—It is typically in the 30–40 age group.

A.3.7 a. F—It is the only hypotensive that is safe in all stages of pregnancy.
b. T—Pregnancy is not advised for 2 years after cessation of treatment.
c. T
d. F—But warfarin does.
e. T

A.3.8 a. F
b. T
c. T
d. T
e. T

Q.3.9   Polycystic ovary disease:

a. Presentation is typically with menorrhagia
b. Breast development is typically delayed
c. There is characteristically excessive androgenic secretion
d. Obesity is typical
e. Hirsutism is a characteristic finding

Q.3.10   Primary dysmenorrhea:

a. The patient is typically nulliparous
b. Retrograde menstruation has been shown to occur
c. The genital tract is typically normal
d. The contraceptive pill is ineffective in relief of pain
e. Sufferers typically have a high neuroticism score.

Q.3.11   Invasive carcinoma of the cervix:

a. Blood-borne metastatic spread is typical
b. Pain is a typical early feature
c. Offensive vaginal discharge is a characteristic presenting feature
d. Survival depends upon early diagnosis
e. It is typically radioresistant

Q.3.12   Endometrial carcinoma:

a. Occurrence is typically in the post-menopausal age group
b. There is an increased incidence in diabetics
c. There is an association with unopposed oestrogen therapy for menopausal symptoms
d. Progestogens have been shown to decrease tumour size
e. It has been shown to have a better prognosis than carcinoma of the cervix

Q.3.13   Secondary amenorrhoea is associated with:

a. The combined oral contraceptive pill
b. Thyrotoxicosis
c. Cimetidine therapy
d. Turner's syndrome
e. Polycystic ovaries

For answers see over

Answers

A.3.9 a. F—It is usually with secondary amenorrhoea and infertility.
      b. F—The breasts are usually well developed.
      c. T—This inhibits maturation of the follicles.
      d. T
      e. T

A.3.10 a. T—Childbirth does not abolish the pain but lessens its severity.
      b. T
      c. T
      d. F—It abolishes ovulation and therefore abolishes pain.
      e. F

A.3.11 a. F—Blood-borne metastatic spread is rare; spread is usually lymphatic.
      b. F—It is a late symptom.
      c. T
      d. T—Survival rates are 81% in stage 1, 60% in stage 2, 30% in stage 3, and 8% in stage 4.
      e. F—Very few tumours are radioresistant.

A.3.12 a. T
      b. T
      c. T
      d. T
      e. T

A.3.13 a. T—But never permanently.
      b. T
      c. F
      d. F—There is an association between Turner's syndrome and primary amenorrhoea.
      e. T

Q.3.14 **The following factors have been shown to predispose to pre-eclampsia:**

a. Multiparity
b. Multiple pregnancy
c. Migraine prior to the pregnancy
d. Family history of pre-eclampsia
e. Diabetes with vascular disease

Q.3.15 **Maternal diabetes has been shown to be associated with the following in pregnancy:**

a. Hydramnios
b. An increased incidence of congenital abnormalities in the foetus
c. An increased rate of deterioration in pre-existing retinopathy
d. Obstructed labour
e. Premature labour

Q.3.16 **The following maternal factors are recognised to be associated with pre-term labour:**

a. Non-smoker
b. High socio-economic group
c. Previous abortion
d. Renal disease
e. Alcohol problems

Q.3.17 **Maternally transmitted infection in the neonate**

a. is typically caused by streptococci
b. has a recognised association with low birth rate
c. is unrelated to the sex of the baby
d. has been shown to be associated with maternal urinary tract infection
e. is typically acquired via the trans-placental route

For answers see over

Answers

A.3.14 a. F—Pre-eclampsia is 15 times commoner in primigravidae than in parous women.
          b. T
          c. T
          d. T—Predisposition may be inherited as a recessive trait.
          e. T—The risk is very high in such cases.

A.3.15 a. T
          b. T—Perinatal mortality is 25–60/1000 deliveries, of which half are due to congenital abnormalities.
          c. T—Therefore there should be increased ophthalmic follow-up.
          d. T—Owing to the association with large babies.
          e. T—There is also an association with unexplained intra-uterine death after 36 weeks' gestation.

A.3.16 a. F—There is an association with smoking.
          b. F—The association is with membership of a low socio-economic group.
          c. T
          d. T
          e. T

A.3.17 a. T—And by E. Coli.
          b. T—There is less immunocompetence.
          c. F—It is commoner in males.
          d. T
          e. F—It is typically acquired during passage through the birth canal.

Q.3.18   The climacteric:

a. The average age of the menopause in the United Kingdom has been shown to be 50 years
b. Demineralisation of bone takes place after the menopause
c. The level of prolactin rises after the last period
d. The severity of flushing has been shown to be related to the level of oestrogen in the blood
e. Clinical studies have shown that the later the menarche the earlier the menopause

Q.3.19   The menarche:

a. The average age of onset in the United Kingdom is 11 years
b. The pubertal growth spurt occurs earlier in girls than in boys
c. Menarche delayed beyond 16 years is an indication for specialist referral
d. The first sign of puberty is the appearance of pubertal hair
e. Puberty is typically delayed in Turner's syndrome

Q.3.20   Atrophic vaginitis:

a. Typically atrophic changes also will occur in the urethral and bladder mucosa
b. Vaginal itching is associated with glycosuria in the majority of cases
c. Local oestrogens have been shown not to be absorbed systematically
d. Changes in pH of the vaginal lining predispose to infection with pathogenic organisms
e. Regular sexual intercourse has been shown to prevent vaginal atrophy

For answers see over

Answers

A.3.18 a. T
  b. T
  c. F—It falls.
  d. F—There is no relationship.
  e. F—Numerous studies have shown no relationship between the two.

A.3.19 a. F—It is 13 years.
  b. T
  c. T
  d. F—The first sign is the accelerated growth spurt.
  e. T—There is also short stature in the full syndrome; the chromosome pattern is XO.

A.3.20 a. T—Such changes give rise to dysuria and frequency.
  b. F—This is a typical symptom of senile vaginitis.
  c. F—Absorption is considerable.
  d. T
  e. T

Q.3.21 Hysterectomy:

    a. It is undertaken more frequently in higher socio-economic groups

    b. In post-menopausal women the ovaries should be removed routinely because they have ceased hormonal production

    c. Premature ovarian failure is more common in women undergoing hysterectomy

    d. The frequency of orgasm has been shown to decrease

    e. Weight gain is a characteristic feature following hysterectomy

Q.3.22 Pelvic inflammatory disease:

    a. After 3 attacks of pelvic infection the probability of tubal occlusion is greater than 50%

    b. The ESR is raised in the majority of patients during an acute episode

    c. It is the most common cause of infertility

    d. It has been shown to present with secondary dysmenorrhoea

    e. At laparoscopy the majority of suspected cases will have inflamed fallopian tubes

Q.3.23 Obstetric ultrasound:

    a. Renal agenesis can be diagnosed by a scan at 18 weeks' gestation

    b. The majority of congenital heart defects can be detected by a routine scan at 30 weeks' gestation

    c. No harmful foetal affects of ultrasound have been shown

    d. Hydrocephaly can be diagnosed at 16 weeks' gestation

    e. Examination at 8 weeks' gestation has been shown to be the most accurate time to verify gestational age

Q.3.24 The following factors would put a patient of 30 weeks' gestation into a high risk category:

    a. Weight gain of 0.1 kg per week

    b. Proteinuria on three occasions in the absence of hypertension or urinary tract infection

    c. Glycosuria on three occasions

    d. Breech presentation

    e. Anaemia

For answers see over

Answers

A.3.21   a. T—It is performed twice as frequently in the highest group as in the others.
   b. F—The ovaries continue with hormonal production after the menopause and therefore should be conserved.
   c. T—Probably owing to disruption of ovarian blood supply at the time of operation.
   d. F—Prospective studies have shown no change.
   e. F—Again, studies have shown no difference.

A.3.22   a. T—It is approximately 75%.
   b. F—It is raised in approximately 40%.
   c. F—It accounts for 20% of infertility.
   d. T
   e. T—60% do so.

A.3.23   a. T
   b. F—A routine scan can only detect whether heart failure is present, unless it is done in a specialised centre.
   c. T
   d. T
   e. F—16 weeks is the most accurate time.

A.3.24   a. T—Anything less than 0.2 kg.
   b. T
   c. T
   d. F—But it would at 36 weeks.
   e. T

Q.3.25   Maternal alcohol consumption and pregnancy:

a. Alcohol histories have been shown to be reliable at antenatal booking
b. A raised maternal γ-glutamyltransferase has been shown to be associated with an increased incidence of congenital abnormality
c. Drinking 14 units of alcohol weekly has been shown to decrease foetal head circumference
d. The foetal alcohol syndrome has been described in people drinking 20 units of alcohol per week
e. A short upper lip is the major diagnostic feature of the foetal alcohol syndrome

Q.3.26   Systemic lupus erythematosus and pregnancy:

a. There is an increased rate of spontaneous abortion
b. An increased rate of hypertension has been shown
c. There is an increased risk of exacerbation of the disease during pregnancy
d. Infertility has been shown to be more common than in non-affected patients
e. Steroid therapy is contra-indicated during and after delivery

Q.3.27   Statistically it has been shown that

a. uncomplicated post-maturity above 42 weeks' gestation is an indication for induction of labour
b. perinatal mortality falls with an increase in the rate of Caesarian sections
c. babies born normally in consultant care have higher Apgar scores than those born normally in general practice care
d. home delivery is safer than hospital delivery for those with low risk factors at the outset of the pregnancy
e. the decrease in perinatal mortality correlates with the increase in the number of hospital deliveries

For answers see over

Answers

A.3.25 a. F—They are never reliable.
b. T
c. T
d. F—Usually over 60 units per week must be consumed.
e. T—Short palpebral fissures are another feature.

A.3.26 a. T
b. T
c. T
d. T
e. F—It needs to be increased during delivery and continued for at least 6 weeks post-confinement in order to prevent relapse.

A.3.27 a. F—Comparison of 2000 induced and spontaneous labours.
b. F—Any obstetric intervention increases perinatal mortality.
c. F—The reverse is true.
d. T
e. F—They have a negative correlation coefficient.

Q.3.28   In a normal pregnancy

    a. the heart remains the same size
    b. the ESR remains normal
    c. the white cell count is decreased
    d. forced expiratory volume decreases
    e. small bowel transit time is decreased

Q.3.29   Amniocentesis:

    a. It has an induced abortion rate of 1%
    b. Blood contamination of the fluid will make cell culture less reliable
    c. A chronic leak of liquor following procedure has been shown to cause flexion deformities of the hip and ankles of the foetus
    d. Hairlip can be diagnosed by amniocentesis
    e. At the maternal age of 38 years the risk of Down's syndrome is greater than the risks of amniocentesis

Q.3.30   First trimester abortions have been shown to be associated with:

    a. Cervical incompetence
    b. Diabetes mellitus
    c. Pre-existing hypertension
    d. Deficiency of progestogens
    e. Hyperthyroidism

For answers see over

Answers

A.3.28   a. F—It enlarges mainly due to dilatation.
          b. F—It is raised well above normal.
          c. F—It is increased.
          d. F—It remains the same.
          e. F—It is increased.

A.3.29   a. T
          b. T—It also makes alpha-fetoprotein estimations less reliable.
          c. T
          d. F—But it can be detected by fetoscopy.
          e. F—At 38 the risk of Down's syndrome is 1/177.

A.3.30   a. F
          b. F
          c. F
          d. F
          e. T

4. Therapeutics

Q.4.1 **The following drugs have been banned by the Sports Council for competitive athletes:**
a. Ibuprofen
b. Coproxamol
c. Pseudoephedrine
d. Sodium cromoglycate
e. Terfenadine

Q.4.2 **Maternal milk secretion is reduced by the following drugs:**
a. Metoclopramide
b. Ethanol
c. Chlorpromazine
d. Bendrofluazide
e. Methyldopa

Q.4.3 **When prescribing a drug for a vomiting patient:**
a. Domperidone is more likely than metoclopramide to cause a dystonic reaction
b. In identical doses domperidone is cheaper than metoclopramide
c. Prochlorperazine is more sedative than metoclopramide
d. Domperidone is available in suppositories, tablets and injection using an F.P.10
e. Metoclopramide has been shown to cause gynaecomastia

Q.4.4 **The following drugs have been shown to cause a rise in blood glucose:**
a. Frusemide
b. Ethanol
c. Aspirin
d. Phenytoin
e. Metronidazole

Q.4.5 **The following drugs have been shown to produce local gastric irritation:**
a. Allopurinol
b. Digoxin
c. Lithium
d. Nitrofurantoin
e. Co-trimoxazole

For answers see over

Answers

A.4.1 a. F—NSAIDs are allowed.
  b. T—Paracetamol is allowed but opiates are not.
  c. T—One must beware as it is contained in cough and cold remedies.
  d. F—But Intal Co is not allowed.
  e. F—Antihistamines are allowed.

A.4.2 a. F—It increase milk production.
  b. T
  c. F—Again, it increases milk production.
  d. T
  e. F—It increases milk production.

A.4.3 a. F—The reverse is true.
  b. F—Domperidone is nearly four times more expensive.
  c. T
  d. F—The injection has been withdrawn because of cardiac arrhythmias.
  e. T

A.4.4 a. T
  b. F—It causes a fall.
  c. F—It causes a fall.
  d. T
  e. T

A.4.5 a. T
  b. F—It is best given on an empty stomach.
  c. T
  d. T
  e. T

Q.4.6 **The following drugs have been shown to interact with alcohol:**

    a. Griseofulvin
    b. Triazolam
    c. Chlorpropamide
    d. Metronidazole
    e. Frusemide

Q.4.7 **Acyclovir:**

    a. It is more active against varicella zoster than herpes simplex
    b. It is active against cytomegalovirus
    c. Drug resistance against herpes simplex has been shown
    d. Dosage levels should be reduced in cases of renal impairment
    e. Teratogenic effects have been shown in humans

Q.4.8 **Theophylline levels are significantly raised by the concurrent use of:**

    a. Allopurinol
    b. Erythromycin
    c. Phenytoin
    d. Cimetidine
    e. Diazepam

Q.4.9 **It has been shown that drug-induced systemic lupus erythematosus may be caused by:**

    a. Phenytoin
    b. Metronidazole
    c. Methyldopa
    d. Chlorpromazine
    e. Combined oral contraceptives

Q.4.10 **Teratogenic effects have been shown for the following drugs:**

    a. Lithium
    b. Diazepam
    c. Heparin
    d. Stilboestrol
    e. Tetanus toxoid vaccine

For answers see over

Answers

A.4.6   a. F
    b. T—Alcohol potentiates its effect.
    c. T—Alcohol potentiates its effect.
    d. T—An "antabuse" reaction occurs.
    e. F

A.4.7   a. F—The opposite is true; hence the need for an increased dose in shingles.
    b. F
    c. T
    d. T—It is excreted largely unchanged by the kidney.
    e. F

A.4.8   a. T—Enzyme inhibition leads to toxicity of theophylline.
    b. T—Enzyme inhibition occurs.
    c. F
    d. T—Enzyme inhibition occurs.
    e. F—But receptor antagonism reduces the effect of diazepam.

A.4.9   a. T
    b. F
    c. F
    d. T
    e. T

A.4.10   a. T—Congenital heart disease has been demonstrated.
    b. T—Orofacial abnormalities may occur.
    c. F—It does not cross the placenta.
    d. T—Abnormalities in the genital tract may occur.
    e. F—But live vaccines cause multiple abnormalities.

Q.4.11   Indomethacin has been shown to

a. cause premature closure of the ductus arteriosus
b. interact with captopril
c. cause seizures in the infant if given to a breast-feeding mother
d. cause weight loss
e. cause confusion in the elderly

Q.4.12   The following drugs have been shown to be effective if administered via the buccal mucosa:

a. Tabs diamorphine
b. Tabs prochlorperazine
c. Nifedipine
d. Buprenorphine
e. Isosorbide dinitrate

Q.4.13   Diamorphine elixir for the relief of pain in terminal patients:

a. Initial sedation typically continues whilst the drug is administered
b. Analgesia is enhanced if cocaine is added
c. Constipation is a characteristic sequel to treatment
d. Dependence occurs rapidly
e. The same amount of pain relief is produced as when the same dose is given via intramuscular injection

Q.4.14   Allopurinol treatment:

a. The rate of excretion of uric acid is increased
b. Ampicillin-type drug rashes are commoner in those receiving treatment with both drugs
c. An NSAID given during the first 3 months will reduce the incidence of breakthrough attacks of pain
d. Dietary restriction of purine-rich foods is advisable
e. Dyspepsia has been shown to occur

For answers see over

Answers

A.4.11   a. T
           b. T
           c. T
           d. T
           e. T

A.4.12   a. T—It avoids first pass metabolism and is highly soluble.
           b. T—Specific buccal formulations are now available.
           c. T—It produces a short-lived high plasma concentration within minutes.
           d. T—First pass metabolism is avoided.
           e. T

A.4.13   a. F—Sedation occurring in the first few days typically wears off, leaving the patient alert.
           b. F—Hallucinations also tend to occur.
           c. T—An aperient should always be added to the treatment regime.
           d. F—Addiction is not a problem.
           e. F—An intramuscular injection is three times more effective than the same oral dose.

A.4.14   a. F—It inhibits the formation of uric acid by blocking the enzyme oxidase.
           b. T
           c. T—This should be routine management.
           d. F
           e. T—Dyspepsia is one of the commonest side-effects.

Q.4.15 Cimetidine

   a. has been shown to have anti-androgenic activity
   b. acts against *Campylobacter pyloris*
   c. interacts with warfarin
   d. has been shown to be as effective in the treatment of reflux oesphagitis as it is in the treatment of peptic ulcer
   e. 800 mg is no cheaper than 40 mg famotidine

Q.4.16 Tolerance of nitrates

   a. is less likely to be induced by transdermal nitrate patches than by buccal glyceryl trinitrate given 8 hourly
   b. is permanent, once developed
   c. has been shown to develop within 48 hours of the start of the treatment
   d. has been shown to be produced more quickly by isosorbide mononitrate than by isosorbide dinitrate
   e. will not be produced by sustained release preparations, if given once daily

Q.4.17 Tamoxifen

   a. has been shown to prolong disease-free intervals in breast cancer
   b. has been shown to be more effective treatment in older women
   c. has hypercalcaemia as a recognised complication
   d. typically causes amenorrhoea in pre-menopausal patients
   e. has been shown to be effective in the treatment of infertility in patients without carcinoma of the breast

Q.4.18 Combined oral contraceptives

   a. are less effective in preventing ectopic pregnancy than in preventing intrauterine pregnancy
   b. inhibit lactation
   c. are contra-indicated if the previous pregnancy was a hydatidiform mole
   d. increase the risk of inflammatory bowel disease
   e. are contra-indicated in paraplegic women

For answers see over

Answers

A.4.15   a. T—It causes gynaecomastia rarely.
         b. F
         c. T—Ranitidine does not.
         d. F—All H_2 antagonists are less effective in the treatment of reflux oesophagitis.
         e. F—It is considerably cheaper (1988: £10 per month).

A.4.16   a. F—The sustained release formulation will produce tolerance.
         b. F—A short nitrate-free period abolishes the effects of tolerance.
         c. T—This is, however, unusual.
         d. F—They both produce it at the same rate.
         e. T—As there is a nitrate-free period.

A.4.17   a. T—But it has not been shown to prolong the length of survival.
         b. T
         c. T—This usually occurs in the first 6 weeks and may be associated with increased bone pain.
         d. T—This is because of its anti-oestrogenic effect.
         e. T

A.4.18   a. F—They stop ovulation and therefore prevent both.
         b. T—They are therefore unsuitable in breast-feeding mothers.
         c. T—Especially if there is still detectable hCG.
         d. T—Therefore they should not be given to patients with established disease.
         e. T—They increase the risk of thrombosis.

Q.4.19   Benzodiazepines:

a. Long acting compounds have been shown to cause more dependency problems than shorter acting compounds
b. Lorazepam has been shown to be an effective anti-emetic in patients receiving chemotherapy
c. On withdrawal, rebound anxiety takes 2 weeks to develop
d. Epileptic seizures have been shown to occur on withdrawal
e. The majority of long-term users will have symptoms of withdrawal

Q.4.20   Influenza vaccine:

a. It is a live vaccine
b. It is contra-indicated in those people who have severe egg allergy
c. Elderly patients in residential homes are considered an "at risk" group by the DHSS
d. Protective levels of antibody will last for 6 months
e. The protective rate in immunised patients approaches 100%

Q.4.21   Malaria prophylaxis:

a. Chloroquine is safe in pregnancy
b. Retinal toxicity is a complication of short-term chloroquine therapy
c. Proguanil has been shown to cause toxic drug eruptions
d. Pyrimethamine—dapsone combination has been shown to cause methaemoglobinaemia
e. Hydroxychloroquinine is equivalent in price to chloroquine

Q.4.22   Clinically significant interactions take place between the following drugs:

a. Indomethacin and haloperidol
b. Antihistamines and chlorpromazine
c. Metoclopramide and haloperidol
d. Phenytoin and chlorpromazine
e. Levodopa and metoclopramide inhibitors

For answers see over

Answers

A.4.19 a. F—The opposite is true.
          b. T—It is as effective as high dose metoclopramide.
          c. F—It can occur within 2 days.
          d. T—Usually with rapid reduction.
          e. F—Approximately 15% are truly addicted.

A.4.20 a. F—Live vaccine is available but not commercially.
          b. T
          c. T
          d. F—They last for 1 year.
          e. F—It is approximately 70%.

A.4.21 a. T
          b. F—It is a complication of long-term therapy. It is recommended that therapy is not continued for longer than 6 years in total.
          c. F—This is a complication of Fansidar, which is no longer recommended.
          d. T
          e. F—Chloroquine is much cheaper.

A.4.22 a. T—Excessive drowsiness has been reported.
          b. T—Chlorpromazine causes potentiation of the sedative effects of the antihistamine.
          c. T—The combination may precipitate movement disorder.
          d. T—The metabolism of phenytoin is inhibited, thus causing toxicity.
          e. T—The plasma concentration of levodopa is increased.

Q.4.23 Calcium antagonists

    a. relax smooth muscle
    b. typically cause a bradycardia
    c. inhibit uterine action
    d. have been shown to be followed by a deterioration in myocardial function if treatment is terminated suddenly
    e. have been shown to have a teratogenic effect

Q.4.24 The following drugs undergo substantial first pass metabolism:

    a. Salbutamol
    b. Imipramine
    c. Aspirin
    d. Theophylline
    e. Propranolol

Q.4.25 Oral hypoglycaemics:

    a. Glibenclamide has a longer half-life than chlorpropamide
    b. Biguanides stimulate insulin release
    c. Sulphonylureas typically encourage weight gain
    d. Chlorpropamide is contra-indicated in the elderly
    e. Metformin has been shown to cause lactic acidosis

Q.4.26 The following have been shown to be beneficial in treating the pruritus associated with advanced malignancy:

    a. Cimetidine
    b. Cholestyramine
    c. Erythromycin
    d. Ibuprofen
    e. Imipramine

For answers see over

Answers

A.4.23 a. T—Not only in arteries but also in other smooth muscle sites.

      b. F—Often a reflex tachycardia occurs due to the fall in blood pressure at the start of therapy; therefore calcium antagonists are often combined with a beta-blocker.

      c. T—They should not be given at the end of the pregnancy.

      d. T—They can precipitate infarction.

      e. F

A.4.24 a. T

      b. T

      c. T

      d. F

      e. T

A.4.25 a. F—The reverse is true.

      b. F—Sulphonylureas stimulate insulin release; biguanides increase peripheral utilisation of glucose and stimulate gluconeogenesis.

      c. T

      d. T—Due to the long half-life accumulation can occur.

      e. T—Although it was commoner with the now discontinued phenformin.

A.4.26 a. T

      b. T—It binds bile salts.

      c. F

      d. F

      e. T

Q.4.27   In the drug treatment of epilepsy:

a. serum carbamazepine levels are increased by phenytoin
b. carbamazepine toxicity has been shown to be produced by concurrent cimetidine therapy
c. phenytoin levels have been shown to be increased by prochlorperazine
d. phenytoin decreases the serum levels of steroids
e. phenytoin levels are decreased by treatment with benzodiazepines

Q.4.28   Inhaler therapy in asthma:

a. Pressurised aerosol inhalers have been shown to have no decrease in side-effects compared with oral therapy
b. Dry powder inhalers require synchronisation of inspiration with operation of the device
c. Dry powder inhalers are cheaper than pressurised aerosol inhalers
d. Inhaled steroid is available in multiple dose dry pressure inhaler
e. Patient compliance is easier to check with dry powder inhalers than with pressurised aerosol inhalers

Q.4.29   Anti-fungals:

a. Imidazole drugs have a broader spectrum than griseofulvin
b. Topical imidazole preparations typically cause an allergic dermatitis if used for more than 2 weeks
c. Oral ketoconazole has been shown to cause hepatitis
d. Topical imidazole preparations are contra-indicated in the first trimester of pregnancy
e. Topical miconazole has been shown to have activity against *Staphylococcus aureus*

For answers see over

Answers

A.4.27 a. F—They are decreased.
  b. T—Such therapy increases serum levels of carbamazepine.
  c. T—They are also increased by chlorpromazine, imipramine and barbiturates.
  d. T
  e. T

A.4.28 a. F
  b. F—The whole rationale of these devices is to remove the need for coordination.
  c. F—They are considerably more expensive.
  d. T—Using diskhalers.
  e. T—It is difficult to check how much is left in an aerosol can.

A.4.29 a. T—They also have a broader spectrum than nystatin and amphotericin B.
  b. F—They rarely cause this reaction; treatment often needs to be prolonged beyond 2 weeks.
  c. T—The risk is 1 in 10000; the chances are greater if treatment is prolonged beyond 2 weeks.
  d. F—They are not contra-indicated at any stage of pregnancy.
  e. T

Q.4.30 Aspirin has been shown to

a. decrease the risk of myocardial infarction in those with a previous cerebrovascular episode

b. reduce the mortality from acute myocardial infarction if given as soon as possible after the occlusion

c. be associated with an increased risk of retinal haemorrhage

d. decrease the incidence of first myocardial infarctions if given prophylactically to a previously healthy population

e. be more effective as a preventative agent in vascular disease if given in a dose of 300 mg/day rather than 160 mg/day

For answers see over

Answers

A.4.30 a. T—There is a 35% decrease in risk.
b. T—Even if thrombolytic therapy is not given concurrently.
c. T—It also increases the risk of cerebral haemorrhage.
d. F—The British study gave inconclusive results.
e. F—No trial has conclusively proved the benefit of one particu-
lar dose; the incidence of side-effects is dose related.

5. Paediatrics

Q.5.1 Non-accidental injury:
a. Toddlers are at greater risk than babies
b. A colour photograph can be submitted as legal evidence
c. Any bruise on a baby under 6 months is a warning sign
d. Case conferences are typically organised by the consultant paediatrician
e. A torn frenulum of the tongue is a warning sign

Q.5.2 The following have been shown to indicate developmental delay:
a. Lack of eye fixation at 6 weeks
b. Not walking at 15 months
c. No definite words by 2 years
d. Not sitting alone at 7 months
e. Not speaking two-word sentences by 3 years

Q.5.3 Children who are being sexually abused have been shown to present with:
a. Self-mutilation
b. Drug abuse
c. Anorexia nervosa
d. Poor school performance
e. Encopresis

Q.5.4 Sudden infant death syndrome
a. is commoner in males than females
b. is commoner in members of a twin pair than in singletons
c. is commoner in the warm months of the year
d. has its peak incidence in the 1–2 year age group
e. is the commonest cause of infant mortality after the perinatal period

For answers see over

Answers

A.5.1 a. F—The reverse is true.
        b. T
        c. T
        d. F—They are usually organised by the senior social worker.
        e. T—But it also occurs in whooping cough.

A.5.2 a. T
        b. F—18 months is the usual age at which concern develops.
        c. T
        d. F—One year is the age of referral.
        e. T

A.5.3 a. T
        b. T
        c. T
        d. T
        e. T

A.5.4 a. T—Most surveys show a slight predominance of male deaths.
        b. T—The rate for a twin is two to five times higher.
        c. F—The peak incidence is in January in the Northern Hemisphere and in July in the Southern Hemisphere.
        d. F—Most cases are in the 2–7 month age group.
        e. T—2 deaths per 1000 births.

Q.5.5 **Meningococcal meningitis:**
   a. If it is suspected, benzylpenicillin should be administered prior to hospital admission
   b. Vaccination is available against all strains of meningococcus
   c. Sensorineural deafness has been shown to be the most common permanent sequela
   d. It has been shown to be more common in those children in contact with cigarette smoke
   e. Rifampicin has been shown to be the treatment of choice for close contacts

Q.5.6 **Gifted children typically have:**
   a. Early loss of primitive reflexes
   b. Early smiling
   c. Early vocalisation
   d. Early appearance of hand regarding
   e. Less sleep than the average baby

Q.5.7 **Typical features of a baby born with congenital rubella syndrome include:**
   a. Nerve deafness
   b. Thrombocytopenia
   c. Patent ductus arteriosus
   d. Optic atrophy
   e. Absence of one of the bones of the forearm

Q.5.8 **Urinary tract infection in children**
   a. is typically symptomless in the pre-school age group
   b. has an equal sex incidence
   c. is associated with failure to thrive
   d. should be investigated after the first bacteriologically proven attack in both sexes
   e. is associated with renal scarring if attacks start after the age of 8 years

For answers see over

Answers

A.5.5 a. T—This may be life saving.
        b. F—Only against groups A and C.
        c. T
        d. T
        e. T

A.5.6 a. T
        b. T
        c. T
        d. T
        e. T

A.5.7 a. T—This is a typical feature of later (12–16 week) infection.
        b. T—It appears shortly after birth and spontaneously recovers.
        c. T
        d. F—Cataract and retinopathy are typical associations.
        e. F

A.5.8 a. T
        b. F—It is commoner in girls.
        c. T
        d. T
        e. F—Scarring is rare in attacks starting after the age of 5 years.

Q.5.9   Coeliac disease

    a. typically presents in the first month of life
    b. has been shown to present with vomiting
    c. has been shown to present with meconium ileus
    d. is associated with secondary lactose intolerance
    e. typically presents with anaemia in later childhood

Q.5.10   The following features would support a diagnosis of grand mal epilepsy in an infant:

    a. Red face during an attack
    b. Cessation of movement without loss of muscle tone
    c. Late loss of consciousness
    d. Complex stereotyped purposeful movements
    e. Eyes deviated upwards and limbs stiff

Q.5.11   Breast-fed infants have a lower incidence of the following when compared with wholly bottle fed infants:

    a. Ischaemic heart disease in later life
    b. Gastroenteritis
    c. Sudden infant death syndrome
    d. Iron deficiency anaemia
    e. Infantile eczema

Q.5.12   Duchenne muscular dystrophy:

    a. Female carriers show typical features
    b. Shoulder muscle weakness appears before leg weakness
    c. Osteoporosis is a typical complicating feature
    d. Those affected show characteristic features by the fifth year of life
    e. Mean I.Q. is lower than in the average population

For answers see over

Answers

A.5.9   a. F—It usually presents after the child has been weaned.
           b. T
           c. F—Meconium ileus suggests cystic fibrosis.
           d. T—This may be the cause of failure to respond to a gluten-free diet.
           e. T—Along with failure to thrive.

A.5.10   a. F—It is associated with breath-holding.
           b. F—This is a feature of petit mal epilepsy or a focal seizure.
           c. F—Again, this is an effect of breath-holding.
           d. F—Tics and focal fits involve such movements.
           e. T

A.5.11   a. F
           b. T
           c. T
           d. F—This is more common in breast-fed children.
           e. T

A.5.12   a. T—Raised creatine phosphokinase and muscle biopsy changes.
           b. F
           c. T—Secondary to immobility.
           d. T—They often appear by the age of 3 years.
           e. T—Mean I.Q. is 20 points lower than the expected value.

Q.5.13   At 6 weeks of age

   a. hip dysplasia is more easy to detect than at birth
   b. if present, squint is detectable
   c. typically the infant should fixate on the face of the examiner
   d. hearing defects are typically detectable
   e. infants who sleep prone have been shown to be more advanced at lifting their heads

Q.5.14   Headache in children:

   a. Migraine has been shown to be the commonest cause of headache in under 5 year olds
   b. Nocturnal headache is an indication for referral
   c. A headache that is present every day starting in the afternoon and continuing until bedtime indicates intracranial pathology
   d. If a cerebral tumour is present, papilloedema is a typical finding on first presentation
   e. Migraine is precipitated by specific foods in the majority of childhood cases

Q.5.15   Nocturnal enuresis:

   a. If wetting also occurs in the day a buzzer alarm is of little value at night
   b. Treatment should commence at the age of $3\frac{1}{2}$ years
   c. The earlier treatment starts, the greater are the chances of success
   d. Fluid restriction in the evening has been shown to be of value
   e. The majority of children are dry after 4 months' treatment with a buzzer alarm

For answers see over

Answers

A.5.13 a. F
          b. T
          c. T—Failure to do so is an indication for referral.
          d. F—They are usually checked for at 7–8 months.
          e. T

A.5.14 a. F—It is rare in under 5 year olds.
          b. T—Especially if the history is of short duration.
          c. F—It is more likely to be due to emotional tension.
          d. T—It is present in the majority of cases at first examination.
          e. F—Only in about 10%.

A.5.15 a. F—Daytime wetting occurs in 10%.
          b. F—Treatment is of little value below 5 years.
          c. F
          d. F
          e. T—80% with a 10% relapse rate.

Q.5.16   Chronic diarrhoea:

a. The presence of recognisable food in the stool has been shown to be associated with cow's milk intolerance
b. Cow's milk intolerance typically resolves by the age of 2 years
c. In cystic fibrosis an abnormal gene is inherited from both parents
d. Faecal fat estimates have been shown to be the single most valuable investigation
e. *Giardia lamblia* has been shown to be the commonest infective cause for prolonged diarrhoea in the United Kingdom

Q.5.17   Appendicitis in children:

a. Perforation is commoner than in adults
b. Constipation is typical
c. Rectal examination should be performed prior to hospital admission
d. Elevation of the white cell count has been shown to be a characteristic feature
e. A 2-year-old child can typically locate the pain with accuracy

Q.5.18   Petit mal epilepsy:

a. Learning problems are typical
b. It characteristically proceeds to grand mal attacks in later life
c. Phenytoin is the drug of choice
d. The EEG appearance is typical
e. Episodes of altered consciousness typically last for more than 1 minute

Q.5.19   Down's syndrome is associated with:

a. Hypothyroidism
b. An increased incidence of leukaemia
c. Syndactyly
d. Flat feet
e. Ventricular septal defects

For answers see over

Answers

A.5.16 a. F—The diagnosis will probably be "toddler" diarrhoea due to failure to chew food.
         b. T
         c. T—Inheritance is autosomal recessive.
         d. F—They are rarely done; a growth chart is the most valuable investigation.
         e. T

A.5.17 a. T—The appendix wall is thinner.
         b. F—Both constipation and diarrhoea may occur.
         c. F—It should be inflicted on a child only once and is best left to the person who will decide whether to operate or not.
         d. F—It is of little significance in children.
         e. F—A child usually can do this at 3 years of age.

A.5.18 a. T—Due to lack of attention.
         b. F—It does so only occasionally.
         c. F—Ethosuximide or sodium valproate is usually the drug of choice.
         d. T
         e. F—They typically last 10-15 seconds.

A.5.19 a. T—The incidence is very high in later life.
         b. T
         c. F
         d. T
         e. T

Q.5.20 In a child with growth failure the following have been shown to indicate that referral to a paediatrician is necessary:

a. Clinical signs of wasting
b. A slowing of the rate of growth
c. Social deprivation
d. Parental short stature
e. Height below the 3rd percentile

Q.5.21 Purpuric rashes in children

a. are most commonly caused by Henoch-Schönlein purpura
b. may indicate idiopathic thrombocytopenic purpura
c. are associated with acute leukaemia
d. typically disappear on pressure
e. in Henoch-Schönlein purpura, are typically associated with proteinuria

Q.5.22 Whooping cough:

a. The incubation period is 7 days
b. The period of infectivity in an untreated child is approximately 4 weeks
c. Bronchiectasis is a typical sequel to the illness in a child under 1 year old
d. Cyanosis during an attack of coughing is an indication for admission to hospital
e. In uncomplicated cases there are no abnormal physical signs

Q.5.23 Benign cardiac murmurs in children have been shown to have the following characteristics:

a. They vary with inspiration
b. They are never diastolic
c. They are altered by change in posture
d. They are typically heard over a limited area of the precordium
e. They are never continuous

For answers see over

Answers

A.5.20   a. T
 b. T—Between two measurements 6 months apart.
 c. T—One third of children will have no physical reason for growth failure, and it may be associated with intellectual and emotional deprivation.
 d. F—Unless associated with other problems.
 e. T—As measured on a Tanner chart.

A.5.21   a. T
 b. T
 c. T
 d. F
 e. T

A.5.22   a. T
 b. T—It is only 2 days if erythromycin is given.
 c. F—It is very rare in developed countries.
 d. T—As is a convulsion.
 e. T

A.5.23   a. T—They are also accentuated by tachycardia.
 b. T—They are always systolic.
 c. T
 d. T
 e. F—A venous hum is continuous.

Q.5.24   Speech delay:

a. It is typically seen in deaf children
b. By the age of 2 years the normal child can join words up into simple sentences
c. Stammering at 2 years of age is an indication for speech therapy
d. A vocabulary of 20 words at 2 years of age indicates speech delay
e. Autism has been shown to present as speech delay

Q.5.25   Breath-holding attacks:

a. They typically occur in the first 6 months of life
b. The presence of cyanosis during an attack invalidates the diagnosis
c. Characteristically clonic movements occur during an attack
d. Sodium valproate has been shown to be of benefit in severe cases
e. Typically there is an attack of screaming before the breath-holding episode

For answers see over

Answers

A.5.24 a. T

b. T—Sentences get longer by about one word for every year of life.

c. F—Lisps and misarticulations are also "normal" at this age.

d. F—At 2 years the extent of the vocabulary can vary from 12 to 200 words.

e. T—Note the lack of eye contact in autistic children.

A.5.25 a. F—Occurrence is typically between 6 months and 18 months.

b. F—Cyanosis is characteristic.

c. F—They are not common but can occur in severe attacks.

d. F—No drug therapy has been shown to be of any value.

e. T

6. Surgery

Q.6.1 Carcinoma of the head of the pancreas:

    a. Serum amylase is typically elevated
    b. It is commoner in males
    c. The gall-bladder is typically palpable
    d. Backache is a typical feature
    e. Jaundice is a characteristic presenting symptom

Q.6.2 Leg ulcers:

    a. Large gravitational ulcers are always painful
    b. Treating superficial infection with antibiotics has been shown to be beneficial
    c. Ulcers caused by arterial disease are typically treated by compression bandaging
    d. In diabetic ulcers the dressing should be left in situ for no more than 1 week
    e. Diuretics have been shown to be of benefit in the treatment of associated oedema

Q.6.3 Following successful renal transplantation

    a. secondary infertility acquired during previous dialysis typically fails to reverse
    b. parathyroidectomy is indicated for dialysis-induced hypercalcaemia
    c. non-contact sport should be discouraged
    d. permanent immunosuppressive therapy will be necessary
    e. anaemia acquired during dialysis fails to reverse

Q.6.4 The following are recognised complications of acute pancreatitis:

    a. Pleural effusion
    b. Hypokalaemia
    c. Characteristic ECG changes
    d. Acute pericarditis
    e. Ureteric obstruction

For answers see over

Answers

A.6.1 a. F
       b. T—It is twice as common in males.
       c. T—It is often so distended that it is visible, according to textbooks.
       d. T
       e. T—The classic presenting symptom is obstructive jaundice.

A.6.2 a. F
       b. F
       c. F
       d. T
       e. F—They are only used to treat oedema of general cause, e.g. congestive cardiac failure.

A.6.3 a. F
       b. T—Hypercalcaemia may fail to reverse.
       c. F—Only sport that may damage a superficially placed kidney should be discouraged.
       d. T
       e. F—It usually reverses within 6 months.

A.6.4 a. T
       b. T
       c. T—ST segment depression and T wave depression.
       d. F
       e. F

Q.6.5 Achalasia of the oesophagus

a. is typically painless
b. typically makes liquids more difficult to swallow than solids
c. characteristically presents with loss of weight as an early symptom
d. has been shown to be pre-malignant
e. typically presents with anaemia

Q.6.6 In peripheral vascular disease

a. the foot pulses typically disappear after exercise in early disease
b. associated leg ulcers are typically painless
c. pain occurring at rest typically affects the calf
d. the site of the claudication pain helps to localise the site of the arterial blockage
e. arterial calcification noted on X-rays is associated with a poor prognosis

Q.6.7 After small bowel resection the following are recognised complications:

a. Gastric ulceration
b. Watery diarrhoea
c. Hypercalcaemia
d. An increased incidence of oxalate stones in the urinary tract
e. Vitamin B_{12} deficiency

Q.6.8 Carcinoma of the colon

a. is the commonest malignancy in the alimentary tract
b. shows a lower incidence in vegetarians than in meat eaters
c. is more likely to occur if there has been a previous ureteric transplant into the sigmoid colon
d. shows a familial distribution
e. shows an increased incidence in those who have had breast cancer

For answers see over

Answers

A.6.5 a. F—The pain often responds to glyceryl trinitrate.
        b. F—Both are affected.
        c. F
        d. T
        e. F

A.6.6 a. T—This is a useful physical sign.
        b. F
        c. F—Typically the toes are affected.
        d. F
        e. F

A.6.7 a. F—Duodenal ulceration is.
        b. T—Usually in ileal resections, as bile salts are not resorbed and act on the colonic mucosa.
        c. F
        d. T—Due to increased colonic absorption.
        e. T—If terminal ileum is removed; it will only respond to B_{12} and not to intrinsic factor.

A.6.8 a. T—It is the second commonest malignancy overall, after lung cancer.
        b. T
        c. T—Possibly owing to nitrates excreted in the urine.
        d. T—10% of children of colorectal cancer patients develop the disease.
        e. T—The incidence is also higher in those who have had carcinoma of the ovary or prostate.

Q.6.9   Coronary artery surgery:

    a. The operative mortality is more than 5%

    b. Patients who have triple vessel disease have been shown to have an improved prognosis following successful surgery

    c. Patients with single vessel disease and stable angina have been shown to have an improved prognosis after successful surgery

    d. the majority of patients are free of angina 1 year after surgery

    e. If angina recurs after surgery, re-operation has been shown to abolish angina in the majority of patients

Q.6.10   Gallstones:

    a. The incidence of gallbladder disease is falling in the United Kingdom

    b. Up to 40% of patients still have symptoms after operation

    c. Cancer of the colon has been shown to be more common after cholecystectomy

    d. The majority of patients with gallstones will have no symptoms

    e. Cancer of the gallbladder has been shown to be a complication of untreated gallstones

Q.6.11   Peptic ulcer surgery:

    a. Recurrent gastic ulcer is an indication for surgical intervention

    b. The incidence of "dumping" is decreased by performing selective vagotomy

    c. The incidence of recurrence of the ulcer has been shown to be higher after selective vagotomy

    d. Diarrhoea has been shown to be more common after vagotomy

    e. B_{12} deficiency has been shown to be a late sequel to surgery

For answers see over

Answers

A.6.9 a. F—It is 1%–2%.
       b. T
       c. F
       d. T—80% or more.
       e. T—It does so in 60%.

A.6.10 a. F—It is rising, especially in men and the young.
       b. T
       c. T
       d. T—More than 50% of gallstones are "silent".
       e. T—100 cholecystectomies need to be performed to prevent one cancer of the gall bladder.

A.6.11 a. T
       b. T
       c. T
       d. T
       e. T

Q.6.12 Cancer of the breast:

a. A G. P. with 2500 patients will see on average two new cases per year
b. The 5-year survival of all patients with breast cancer is less than 50%
c. Alpha-fetoprotein is typically raised above normal
d. Surgery has been shown to improve survival rates more than radiotherapy
e. The incidence has been shown to be less in women who have had previous bilateral oopherectomy for non-malignant disease

Q.6.13 Irritable bowel syndrome:

a. Rectal bleeding is a recognised feature
b. The incidence of colonic carcinoma has been shown to be increased
c. The abdominal pain is typically related to the ingestion of food
d. The pain is typically in the right iliac fossa
e. The typical presenting age is above 50 years

Q.6.14 Anal disease:

a. The pain of an anal fissure is typically relieved by defaecation
b. Anal fissures typically occur in the mid-line
c. Bleeding is not a typical feature of anal fissure
d. Squamous carcinoma is typically painful at a late stage
e. Pruritus ani is typically associated with haemorrhoids

Q.6.15 Testicular torsion:

a. Surgery should be performed within 4 h if the testis is to remain viable
b. Pus in the first voided urine makes a diagnosis of torsion incorrect
c. Doppler blood flow tests show an increased blood flow to the testis in torsion
d. The patient is typically under 18 years of age
e. Torsion typically presents with a more acute onset than epididymitis

For answers see over

Answers

A.6.12
  a. T—Out of a total of ten new cancers per year.
  b. F—But it is only 57%.
  c. F—It is raised in cancer of liver, testis, ovary, pancreas, lung, stomach and colon.
  d. F
  e. T

A.6.13
  a. F—It indicates some other pathological condition.
  b. F—There is no association.
  c. T
  d. T
  e. F—It typically presents in young adults.

A.6.14
  a. F—It usually continues for 1–2 h after defaecation.
  b. T—They usually occur posteriorly.
  c. F—It is, but another pathological condition can also be present.
  d. F—It is typically painful at an early stage.
  e. T

A.6.15
  a. T
  b. T—This is characteristic of epididymitis.
  c. F—The flow is decreased in torsion and increased in epididymitis
  d. T
  e. T

7. ENT

Q.7.1 Otosclerosis:

a. Deafness is sensorineural
b. Progress of the condition has been shown to be accelerated by oral contraceptive therapy
c. Presentation is typically unilateral
d. It is typically a familial condition
e. An association with vertigo has been shown

Q.7.2 Criteria for diagnosing Meniere's disease include:

a. Complete recovery from vertigo between attacks
b. A raised ESR above the normal level
c. Fluctuating sensorineural hearing loss
d. Tinnitus
e. A feeling of fullness in the affected ear

Q.7.3 Acoustic neuroma:

a. It is characterised by progressive unilateral deafness
b. Vertigo occurring early in the illness is typically progressive
c. The facial nerve is typically affected at an early stage
d. It is associated with trigeminal neuralgia
e. Audiometric tests produce a characteristic pattern of hearing loss

Q.7.4 Benign paroxysmal positional vertigo

a. is associated with a previous recent history of head injury
b. typically resolves spontaneously
c. is the commonest cause of vertigo
d. typically involves prolonged attacks
e. is characteristically induced by change of position

Q.7.5 Erosive cholesteatoma:

a. It is associated with short episodes of vertigo
b. Absence of discharge excludes the diagnosis
c. A minimal hearing loss excludes the diagnosis
d. A wet central perforated drum is characteristic
e. It is associated with the development of meningitis

For answers see over

Answers

A.7.1 a. F—Conductive deafness occurs due to fixation of the footplate of the stapes.
        b. T—It is also accelerated in pregnancy.
        c. F—It is slowly progressive, becoming bilateral.
        d. T
        e. T—Similar to the association between Meniere's disease and vertigo.

A.7.2 a. T
        b. F—There is no diagnostic test.
        c. T
        d. T
        e. T

A.7.3 a. T—In cases of bilateral loss think of neurofibromatosis.
        b. F—Vertigo which occurs early, often remits.
        c. F—Sensory and secretomotor fibres are more often affected.
        d. T—Usually when the tumour is more advanced.
        e. F—There are no typical changes.

A.7.4 a. T—It usually occurs within a few days of the injury.
        b. T—Usually within 6 months.
        c. T
        d. F—It usually only lasts a few seconds.
        e. T

A.7.5 a. T—Vertigo and unsteadiness in the course of chronic middle ear disease are worrying.
        b. F—If discharge is present it may be minimal or profuse but is usually foul smelling.
        c. F
        d. F— Erosive cholesteatoma is associated with an attico-antral perforation.
        e. T

Q.7.6   Chronic otitis externa

a. is typically associated with hearing loss
b. is typically unilateral
c. is associated with seborrhoeic dermatitis
d. is associated with psoriasis
e. is best treated with systemic antibiotics

Q.7.7   Tinnitus has been shown to be associated with:

a. Anxiety
b. Occupational hearing loss
c. Otosclerosis
d. Meniere's disease
e. Paget's disease

Q.7.8   Mastoiditis is suggested by the following events during a course of acute otitis media:

a. Headache on the side of the affected ear
b. Normal bony trabeculae on X-ray
c. Deafness
d. Swelling posterior to the ear
e. Abrupt cessation of the earache

Q.7.9   Secretory otitis media in children:

a. Resolution occurs without treatment in the majority of cases
b. Typically there is a history of preceding acute inflammatory otitis media
c. Radial blood vessels of the eardrum exclude the diagnosis
d. Pain in the ear excludes the diagnosis
e. The eardrum is typically concave

Q.7.10   Pain may be referred to the ear from:

a. The parotid gland
b. The posterior one-third of the tongue
c. The temperomandibular joint
d. C2 and C3 nerve roots
e. The pyriform fossa

For answers see over

Answers

A.7.6 a. F
         b. F—It is usually bilateral.
         c. T
         d. T
         e. F—Aural toilet is the treatment of choice.

A.7.7 a. T
         b. T
         c. T
         d. T
         e. T

A.7.8 a. T
         b. F
         c. F
         d. T
         e. F

A.7.9 a. T
         b. F
         c. F—This is a characteristic appearance.
         d. F—Typically the pain is of short duration and is not distressing.
         e. T—It is also opaque.

A.7.10 a. T—Vth nerve.
          b. T—IXth nerve.
          c. T—Vth nerve.
          d. T
          e. T—Xth nerve.

8. Dermatology

Q.8.1 **The following are recognised causes of blistering eruptions:**

   a. Staphylcoccal skin infections
   b. Dermatitis herpetiformis
   c. Pemphigoid
   d. Hand, foot and mouth disease
   e. Scabies

Q.8.2 **The following have been shown to be associated with malignancy:**

   a. Acanthosis nigricans
   b. Tylosis
   c. Dermatitis herpetiformis
   d. Pemphigus
   e. Dermatomyositis

Q.8.3 **Erythema nodosum is a recognised feature of:**

   a. Sulphonamide therapy
   b. Sarcoidosis
   c. Crohn's disease
   d. Hodgkin's disease
   e. Streptococcal sore throat

Q.8.4 **Genital warts:**

   a. They are always sexually transmitted
   b. The wife of a patient with penile warts should have annual cytology
   c. Podophyllin paint can be used with safety during pregnancy
   d. Barrier methods of contraception are recommended until infection has resolved
   e. Contact tracing is recommended

For answers see over

Answers

A.8.1 a. T—Especially in very young babies.
      b. T—Classically it is very itchy.
      c. T—In the elderly.
      d. T
      e. T—It can cause vesicles around the wrist and fingers.

A.8.2 a. T—70% of cases of acanthosis nigricans are associated with gastro-intestinal malignancy.
      b. T—It is associated with carcinoma of the oesophagus.
      c. F—But it is associated with jejunal villous atrophy and coeliac disease.
      d. F
      e. T—Approximately 15% of patients have a neoplasm, usually of the breast or ovary; treatment of the primary often cures the dermatomyositis.

A.8.3 a. T
      b. T
      c. T
      d. T
      e. T—This is the commonest cause in the United Kingdom; the commonest cause worldwide is lepromatous leprosy.

A.8.4 a. F—But they usually are.
      b. T
      c. F—It is toxic to the foetus.
      d. T
      e. T

Q.8.5 **Treatment of acne vulgaris with isotretinoin:**

  a. Pregnancy should be avoided for 6 months after cessation of treatment
  b. Fasting lipids should be checked monthly during the treatment
  c. It should be reserved for nodulocystic acne
  d. Liver function tests remain normal
  e. Eczema is a recognised side-effect of the treatment

Q.8.6 **Malignant melanoma:**

  a. The histological stage of the disease determines the treatment
  b. People with fair hair and blue eyes are at risk
  c. The incidence is remaining stationary
  d. Survival rates are independent of tumour thickness
  e. An increased incidence has been shown in the relatives of patients with a melanoma

Q.8.7 **Psoriasis:**

  a. Early onset is associated with a better prognosis
  b. It can present at any age
  c. The Koebner phenomenon is a characteristic association
  d. NSAIDs have been shown to prevent relapse
  e. PUVA treatment is associated with the subsequent development of skin cancers

Q.8.8 **Skin tumours:**

  a. Kerato-acanthoma typically occurs on light-exposed skin
  b. Bowen's disease typically changes to an invasive carcinoma if not treated
  c. Pyogenic granulomas are typically malignant
  d. Solar keratoses have malignant potential
  e. Epidermoid cysts have been shown to follow severe acne

For answers see over

Answers

A.8.5 a. F—Avoidance for 1 month is recommended.
        b. T—Hyperlipidaemia is common.
        c. T
        d. F—Abnormalities are common and tests should be performed regularly.
        e. T—It can be severe.

A.8.6 a. T
        b. T
        c. F—It is increasing rapidly.
        d. F—The thinner the lesion, the greater the chances of survival
        e. T

A.8.7 a. F—The earlier the onset, the worse the outlook.
        b. T—Females have an earlier age of onset.
        c. T—Lesions develop in skin which has already been damaged.
        d. F—They are associated with exacerbation, as are lithium, beta-blockers, and antimalarials.
        e. T—PUVA, psoralen plus ultra-violet A.

A.8.8 a. T—It will almost invariably disappear spontaneously.
        b. F—This is a rare complication.
        c. F—They erupt rapidly at the site of injury or infection.
        d. T—Although this potential is low.
        e. T—They are consequently most common on the head, neck and trunk.

Q.8.9 **The following skin conditions which occur in pregnancy will typically remit after delivery:**
 a. Pruritis
 b. Spider naevi
 c. Chloasma
 d. Hirsutism
 e. Telogen effluvium

Q.8.10 **Scarring of the scalp has been shown to occur in alopecia due to:**
 a. Fungal infection
 b. Discoid lupus erythematosus
 c. Lichen planus
 d. Alopecia areata
 e. Trichotillomania

Q.8.11 **The nails have been shown to be affected in:**
 a. Treatment with chloroquine
 b. Cirrhosis
 c. Alopecia areata
 d. Peripheral lymphoedema
 e. Cystic fibrosis

Q.8.12 **Pemphigus:**
 a. The blisters characteristically itch
 b. Oral lesions are typical
 c. Treatment with steroids is life-saving
 d. The blisters typically rupture easily
 e. The prognosis is better than that of pemphigoid

Q.8.13 **Vitiligo:**
 a. There is an association with Addison's disease
 b. It is typically symmetrical
 c. Sun exposure has been shown to help repigmentation
 d. Spontaneous improvement is typical
 e. Topical steroids characteristically aid repigmentation

For answers see over

Answers

A.8.9 a. T
          b. T
          c. F
          d. T
          e. F

A.8.10 a. T
          b. T
          c. T
          d. F
          e. F

A.8.11 a. T—Blue nails.
          b. T—Clubbing and opaque nails.
          c. T—Pitting.
          d. T—Yellow nails
          e. T—Clubbing.

A.8.12 a. F—Pemphigoid itches.
          b. T
          c. F—Mortality is high despite steroids.
          d. T
          e. F

A.8.13 a. T—Both have an auto-immune basis although Addison's disease is more typically associated with increased pigmentation.
          b. T—Unilateral areas are rare.
          c. F—Blistering easily occurs and total sun-block should be used.
          d. F—It rarely occurs.
          e. F—They do so in only a very few cases.

Q.8.14   The following statements are true:

    a. Granuloma annulare has been shown to be associated with diabetes

    b. Pyoderma gangrenosum has been shown to be associated with Crohn's disease

    c. Dermatitis herpetiformis is associated with an increased risk of small bowel lymphoma

    d. Necrobiosis lipoidica is characteristically found in known diabetics

    e. Chloasma is associated with oral contraceptive therapy

Q.8.15   Rosacea:

    a. Women are more commonly affected than men

    b. It is associated with conjunctivitis

    c. An auto-immune origin has been shown

    d. "Blackheads" are a typical feature

    e. Topical steroids have been shown to be of benefit

Q.8.16   Cryotherapy with liquid nitrogen:

    a. It has been shown to be suitable treatment for seborrhoeic keratosis

    b. It is contra-indicated for treatment of molluscum contagiosum

    c. Hypopigmentation is a recognised complication

    d. Blistering has been shown to be reduced by the use of strong steroid creams

    e. Painful blisters imply secondary infection

Q.8.17   Erysipelas

    a. is characteristically tender

    b. is excluded by the appearance of vesicles

    c. affects deeper layers of the skin than cellulitis

    d. is always due to streptococcus

    e. has been shown to be associated with cavernous sinus thrombosis if it occurs on the face

For answers see over

Answers

A.8.14 a. T—Typically in women under 30 years of age.

b. T—Association with ulcerative colitis and rheumatoid arthritis has also been shown.

c. T—Most have malabsorption.

d. F—40%–60% of patients with necrobiosis lipoidica will develop diabetes but only 0.3% of patients with known diabetes will develop the condition.

e. T—But it is more typically associated with pregnancy.

A.8.15 a. T

b. T—Often associated with a conjunctivitis which is sensitive to light.

c. F

d. F—They are typical of acne vulgaris.

e. F—They should not be used as they increase skin erythema.

A.8.16 a. T

b. F

c. T—So is hyperpigmentation.

d. T—By a single dose after the treatment.

e. F—They should be burst with a sterile needle and dry dressing applied.

A.8.17 a. T—It is well defined and not oedematous.

b. F—Vesicles are common.

c. F—The reverse is true.

d. F—Staphylococci, *Klebsiella* and *Haemophilus* are all causative organisms.

e. T

Q.8.18 **Pustular psoriasis:**
   a. Typically the hands and feet are affected
   b. An association with cigarette smoking has been shown
   c. The pustules are typically due to secondary infection
   d. Evidence of psoriasis on other parts of the body is characteristically found
   e. It is associated with mouth ulcers

Q.8.19 **The following conditions are typically symmetrical:**
   a. "Mongolian" spots
   b. Spider naevi
   c. Discoid lupus erythematosus
   d. Alopecia areata
   e. Dermatomyositis

Q.8.20 **Hyperthyroidism is associated with the following skin changes:**
   a. Pre-tibial myxoedema
   b. Rapid growth of nails
   c. Palmar erythema
   d. Thinning of scalp hair
   e. Facial flushing

For answers see over

Answers

A.8.18   a. T
             b. T
             c. F—The pustules are sterile.
             d. F—HLA patterns indicate that they may be separate diseases.
             e. F

A.8.19   a. F
             b. F
             c. T
             d. F
             e. T

A.8.20   a. T
             b. T—In hypothyroidism they are brittle and slow growing.
             c. T
             d. T—In hypothyroidism the skin is also coarse.
             e. T

9. Ophthalmology

Q.9.1 Myopia:

a. It has been shown to be due to excessive reading
b. It typically occurs below the age of 6 years
c. Changes in visual acuity typically stop in the late teens
d. Lens opacities are commoner in later life
e. Contact lenses will affect the natural history of the condition in adults

Q.9.2 Cataracts:

a. Diabetic cataracts typically progress more rapidly than those in non-diabetics
b. Surgery is more successful if performed at an early age.
c. There is an increased risk of retinal detachment after cataract surgery
d. Patients are typically hospitalised for 10 days or more for removal of a cataract
e. Binocular vision is lost after a lens implant

Q.9.3 Corneal injury:

a. If a penetrating wound is suspected, instillation of local anaesthetic is contra-indicated
b. A round pupil indicates that penetration of the cornea has not occurred
c. Retained intra-ocular foreign bodies have been shown to cause blindness many years after the injury
d. Superficial corneal abrasions are typically symptom-free 48 h after appropriate treatment
e. Local anaesthetic delays healing of a superficial abrasion

Q.9.4 Squint in children:

a. Referral should be delayed until the cooperation of the child is possible
b. The primary aim of treatment is to achieve good binocular vision
c. Hypermetropia is a characteristic finding
d. Surgery for the squint typically corrects amblyopia
e. A squint which alternates from eye to eye will have a worse prognosis than a squint affecting only one eye

For answers see over

Answers

A.9.1 a. F—This is a common misconception.
        b. F—It rarely occurs below 6 years; peak incidence is at 11 years.
        c. T
        d. F—But secondary degeneration of the retina can occur.
        e. F—However, if young children are not prescribed spectacles they may not reach their full potential visually.

A.9.2 a. T
        b. F—However, early assessment allows the condition of the retina to be evaluated accurately.
        c. T—But it is less after an extracapsular extraction.
        d. F—Modern surgical techniques have led to hospital stays of 2–3 days, and in the United States, to day case surgery.
        e. F

A.9.3 a. F
        b. F—The pupil is usually oval and sluggish but a round pupil does not exclude penetration.
        c. T—X-rays are thus important if a foreign body is suspected.
        d. T—Persistence of pain beyond 48 h may indicate complications.
        e. T

A.9.4 a. F—Referral should be made by 6 months.
        b. T—With satisfactory cosmetic appearance and good visual acuity.
        c. T
        d. F—Ideally surgery should be performed once the visual acuity matches the good eye.
        e. F

Q.9.5 **Acute glaucoma:**
a. If it is suspected, a miotic should be instilled prior to referral
b. Headaches are typical
c. It has been shown to cause abdominal pain
d. Haloes around lights are typically coloured
e. A glaucomatous pupil is typically larger than the other pupil

Q.9.6 **Contact lenses:**
a. They are contra-indicated in patients with hay fever
b. They have been shown to cause corneal vascularisation
c. They have been shown to be of more use in those with large refractive error
d. They are contra-indicated in patients who require regular eye drops
e. Sub-conjunctival haemorrhage is a typical feature of hard lens use

Q.9.7 **Retinal detachment**
a. typically occurs in patients who have previously had congenital cataracts
b. becomes bilateral in the majority of cases
c. may be followed by improvement in visual acuity up to 18 months after surgery
d. has been shown to be the presenting feature of a malignant melanoma
e. characteristically occurs without warning

Q.9.8 **Sudden loss of vision has been shown to occur in:**
a. Tobacco amblyopia
b. Retinal vein occlusion
c. Cranial arteritis
d. Retrobulbar neuritis
e. Hysteria

For answers see over

Answers

A.9.5 a. T—It will do no harm and may save vision.
        b. T
        c. T—Nausea and vomiting are other symptoms.
        d. T—They are often best described as rainbows by patients.
        e. T—It is also more sluggish in the response to light.

A.9.6 a. F
        b. T—This is a complication of long-term use.
        c. T—They are usually more acceptable than high power glasses.
        d. F—Soft lenses cause problems but hard lenses do not.
        e. F—It is no commoner in hard lens wearers.

A.9.7 a. T
        b. F—Only 10% of cases become bilateral.
        c. T
        d. T
        e. F—Floaters and flashes in the eye often herald a detachment.

A.9.8 a. F—Loss is insidious.
        b. T
        c. T—Hence the need for urgent steroids.
        d. T—But it is usually reversible.
        e. T

Q.9.9   Blind registration benefits include:

a. A talking book
b. Mobility allowance
c. Extra income
d. A reduced fee for the television licence
e. A free radio

Q.9.10   Senile macular degeneration:

a. Central scotoma is typically present
b. Alteration in image size is a recognised feature
c. Fluoroscein angiograpy is diagnostic
d. Photophobia has been shown to occur
e. Photopsia is typically found

Q.9.11   Central retinal artery occlusion

a. is associated with a carotid bruit in the majority of cases
b. is associated with hypertension in the majority of cases
c. is characteristically followed by recovery of visual function
d. has been shown to be associated with hyperlipidaemia
e. has been shown to be associated with mitral valve prolapse

Q.9.12   Acute allergic conjunctivitis:

a. Eosinophils are characteristically present in the secretions
b. The eye typically feels "sticky"
c. Crusts typically appear on the eyelids
d. Onset is typically rapid
e. The mucosa shows characteristic appearances

Q.9.13   The following eyedrops are painful when initially instilled into a normal eye:

a. Fluorescein
b. Benoxinate
c. Rose bengal
d. Amethocaine
e. Chloramphenicol

For answers see over

Answers

A.9.9 a. T
      b. F—Blind people have great difficulty getting the allowance but can obtain a disabled badge for a relative's car
      c. T
      d. T
      e. T

A.9.10 a. T
      b. T—Image size is usually decreased but can be increased.
      c. T
      d. T
      e. T

A.9.11 a. F—The figure is 14%–18%.
      b. T—Hypertension occurs in approximately 57%.
      c. F—Only 20% have a limited recovery.
      d. T—15%–30%.
      e. T—34%.

A.9.12 a. T
      b. F—It feels itchy, not sticky.
      c. F—Crusts appear in acute infection.
      d. T
      e. T—"Cobblestone mucosa".

A.9.13 a. F
      b. T
      c. T
      d. T
      e. F

Q.9.14   **Acute optic neuritis**

    a. typically gives a central scotoma
    b. is painless in the majority of cases
    c. typically recurs in the majority of patients
    d. is a forerunner to multiple sclerosis in 50% of patients
    e. is typically associated with profuse retinal haemorrhages

Q.9.15   **When considering the ocular problems of diabetics:**

    a. The finding of persistent albuminuria is typically associated with retinopathy
    b. Retinopathy has been shown to progress more rapidly during pregnancy
    c. The incidence of blindness has decreased since the advent of laser photocoagulation
    d. Macular oedema is a recognised finding
    e. Laser photocoagulation requires a general anaesthetic

For answers see over

Answers

A.9.14 a. T
         b. F—Approximately 75% of patients have peri-orbital pain which is worse on eye movement.
         c. F—There is recurrence in either eye in about 20% of patients.
         d. T
         e. F

A.9.15 a. T—Both are micro-angiopathic conditions.
         b. T
         c. T
         d. T
         e. F

10. *Law/Ethics*

Q.10.1 The following groups of patients are exempt from prescription charges:

a. Hypertensives
b. Thyrotoxics
c. Asthmatics
d. Rheumatoid arthritics
e. Men aged 60 years who have retired on grounds of ill health

Q.10.2 The following allowances are paid to patients independent of a means test:

a. Maternity grant
b. Attendance allowance
c. Mobility allowance
d. Funeral costs grant
e. Milk and vitamins to expectant and nursing mothers

Q.10.3 The General Medical Council will consider action against a doctor for professional misconduct if he

a. issues an N.H.S. prescription to a private patient
b. is banned from driving by the courts for drinking and driving
c. accepts financial rewards from his N.H.S. patients
d. prescribes an anabolic steroid to a competitive athelete
e. comments adversely on the competence of another doctor to a patient

Q.10.4 Ethical principles dictate that a doctor

a. should divulge the HIV positivity of a patient to the patient's spouse
b. should divulge details of suspected child abuse to a social worker without the parent's consent
c. report a colleague for unprofessional conduct
d. obtain the patients' consent before notifying an infectious disease
e. has the absolute right to determine to whom a patient should be referred for a second opinion

For answers see over

Answers

A.10.1 a. F
        b. F
        c. F
        d. F
        e. F

A.10.2 a. F—The patients must be in receipt of income support or family credit.
        b. T
        c. T
        d. F—The patient must be receiving income support, family credit or housing benefit.
        e. F—The patient must be receiving income support.

A.10.3 a. T
        b. T
        c. T
        d. T
        e. T

A.10.4 a. T—According to recent GMC guidelines.
        b. T—The health and welfare of the child are paramount.
        c. T
        d. F
        e. F—This is the patient's right.

Q.10.5 **Current employment legislation states that a general practice with more than five employees must legally provide them with:**

a. A job description
b. An accident report book
c. Paid time off to attend a hospital appointment with their son/daughter
d. A written contract of employment
e. Paid time off to attend trade union meetings

Q.10.6 **The DVLC will consider withdrawing the licence of a car driver who has:**

a. Bilateral severe deafness
b. A single recent epileptic fit
c. A visual acuity of 6/60 in one eye and 6/9 in the other after correction
d. Unstable angina provoked by emotion
e. Diabetes maintained by diet alone

Q.10.7 **Following the Gillick case the General Medical Council has ruled that a doctor:**

a. needs the consent of the parents if the pregnancy of a girl under 16 years of age is to be terminated
b. has the discretion to inform the parents that a girl under 16 years of age has consulted him requesting a termination even if he decides not to carry out the therapeutic abortion
c. needs the consent of the parents to prescribe an oral contraceptive for a girl under 16 years of age
d. has the right to inform the parents that a girl under 16 years of age has consulted him requesting the oral contraceptive
e. has the right to assess the child's maturity and ability to understand the treatment before prescribing the oral contraceptive

For answers see over

Answers

A.10.5 a. F
           b. T
           c. F
           d. T
           e. F

A.10.6 a. F
           b. T
           c. F
           d. T
           e. F

A.10.7 a. F—He should try to persuade her to inform her parents.
           b. T
           c. F
           d. T
           e. T—This is the basis of the guidance.

Q.10.8 **Doctors and the law:**

    a. A doctor must disclose all available medical facts about a death to the coroner/procurator fiscal

    b. The Road Traffic Act obliges doctors to reveal the identity of persons treated in a road traffic accident to a police officer

    c. If a doctor fails to reveal the identity of a patient when ordered to by a magistrate, he will be in contempt of court

    d. A doctor must divulge information about criminal abortion even without the patient's consent

    e. The notes pertaining to a private patient are the legal property of that patient

Q.10.9 **Therapeutic abortion:**

    a. It is legally allowed to take place in any hospital, N.H.S. or private

    b. If it is necessary to save life a second medical opinion is no longer needed

    c. It must be notified to the Chief Medical Officer within 7 days of the termination

    d. Consent from the husband is legally required if he is living with his wife

    e. Certificates must be preserved for 3 years after the procedure

Q.10.10 **The following are notifiable to the Health and Safety Executive:**

    a. Leptospirosis in water board workers

    b. Decompression sickness in divers

    c. Vibration white finger in those using power tools

    d. Urinary tract cancer in aniline dye workers

    e. Mesothelioma in those who have worked with asbestos

For answers see over

Answers

A.10.8   a. T
              b. T
              c. T
              d. F
              e. F—They are the property of the doctor.

A.10.9   a. F—Private hospitals must be licensed.
              b. T
              c. T
              d. F
              e. T

A.10.10   a. T
              b. T
              c. T
              d. T
              e. T

11. *Epidemiology/Research*

Q.11.1 **When evaluating a report of a clinical trial:**

a. Results are invalid if the trial is not of double-blind construction

b. Inadequate sample size has been shown to produce false-positives and false-negatives

c. Withdrawal of patients from a trial by the investigator may be a cause of bias

d. If randomisation is conducted properly, chance differences are inevitable

e. Control and treatment groups must be equivalent in size

Q.11.2 **Ethical considerations in a clinical trial stipulate that**

a. verbal consent is adequate

b. a patient is unable to withdraw once entered into a trial

c. risks and benefits *must* be made known to the patient

d. there must be provision for medically induced injury

e. ethical committees can withhold approval if there is excessive financial incentive

Q.11.3 **Cigarette smoking in the United Kingdom:**

a. The prevalence of cigarette smoking in women is declining.

b. The prevalence of cigarette-related lung cancer is declining in women

c. Smokers remain the majority group in the male unskilled socio-economic group

d. Smoking is more common in schoolgirls than schoolboys

e. The proportion of schoolchildren who smoke is declining

Q.11.4 **Alcohol consumption:**

a. At the age of 15 years the majority of boys drink alcohol regularly on at least a weekly basis

b. There has been a reduction in the number of heavy drinkers during the last decade

c. Alcohol consumption has increased in women

d. Relaxation of alcohol legislation in Scotland has led to an increase in the amount of alcohol consumed in that country

e. The number of people who are moderate drinkers has increased in the last 5 years

For answers see over

Answers

A.11.1 a. F—Single-blind construction is often adequate.
        b. T
        c. T
        d. T
        e. T

A.11.2 a. F—Written consent is needed.
        b. T
        c. T
        d. T
        e. T

A.11.3 a. T—Since 1984 it has declined.
        b. F—It is increasing, reflecting increased smoking habits of women in the 1960's and 1970's.
        c. F—They are now in the minority.
        d. T—The rates are 12% in girls under 16 years and 7% in boys of the same age.
        e. T—It was 10% in 1986 and 13% in 1984.

A.11.4 a. T—52% do so.
        b. T—From 25% of drinkers to 20% since 1978.
        c. T—Mainly in the frequent light drinker category.
        d. F—It is unchanged.
        e. F—It has remained the same: 14%–15%.

Q.11.5 Road traffic accidents:

a. The compulsory wearing of seat belts has reduced the number of fatal accidents by more than 200 per year
b. Compliance with seat belt legislation is greater than 90%
c. The United Kingdom has the lowest death rate for road traffic accidents in Europe
d. Injuries are more likely to occur on a motorway than a trunk road
e. The death rate for road traffic accidents in 1986 was the lowest for 60 years

Q.11.6 The following are true:

a. The prevalence tells how often a situation occurs
b. The incidence tells how common is a situation
c. The specificity of a test is the probability of a negative test given the absence of the condition
d. The sensitivity of a test is the probability of the test being positive in somebody with the condition
e. The reliability of a test is defined as the relevance of the test to the activities being treated

Q.11.7 Retrospective and prospective studies:

a. Retrospective research studies are typically more biased than prospective studies
b. Retrospective research projects are typically quicker than prospective ones
c. The information gathered in a retrospective study is typically of a more definable quality than that gathered in a prospective study
d. Cause and effect relationships are more identifiable in prospective studies
e. Prospective studies typically cost less than retrospective studies

For answers see over

Answers

A.11.5 a. T
        b. T—95%.
        c. T—9.4/100 000 population.
        d. F—They are 3.8 times more common on an A road than on a motorway
        e. T

A.11.6 a. F—The incidence does this.
        b. F—The prevalence does this.
        c. T
        d. T
        e. F—This is the validity; reliability is the ability of a test to produce the same result when repeated under identical conditions.

A.11.7 a. T
        b. T
        c. F—The reverse is true.
        d. T
        e. F—The reverse is true.

Q.11.8   Research protocols typically contain:

    a. Cost estimates
    b. Curriculum vitae of the research worker
    c. References
    d. A review of literature
    e. Details of statistical methods to be used

Q.11.9   Epidemiology of cancer in the United Kingdom:

    a. The incidence of cancer of the stomach has declined in the last 90 years
    b. Deaths from cancer of the oesophagus are decreasing
    c. Pancreatic carcinoma is more frequent in lifelong non smokers
    d. Cancer of the cervix uteri is increasing in women under 35 years of age
    e. Cancer of the testis is rare in black men

Q.11.10   The normal distribution:

    a. A normal curve is bimodal
    b. The mean and the mode are identical
    c. Haemoglobin levels typically show a normal distribution
    d. The mode is the most frequently occurring value
    e. The standard deviation is the square of the variance

For answers see over

Answers

A.11.8   a. T
           b. T
           c. T
           d. T
           e. T

A.11.9   a. T—It used to be the commonest cancer worldwide, but there has been a dramatic decline in incidence throughout the world.
           b. F—They are increasing, especially in the younger age groups.
           c. F—It is much commoner in smokers.
           d. T—Despite screening.
           e. T—The rate is increasing in the United Kingdom, mainly in higher socio-economic groups.

A.11.10   a. F—It is bell-shaped.
            b. T
            c. T
            d. T
            e. F—It is the square root of the variance.

12. Practice Organisation

Q.12.1 **When carried out within general practice the following activities can be considered examples of secondary prevention:**

a. Supervision of diabetics
b. Hypertensive case finding
c. Education of cigarette smokers
d. Obesity clinics
e. Cervical smear clinics

Q.12.2 **Practice staff will qualify for reimbursement only if engaged in one or more of the following duties:**

a. Dispensing
b. Cleaning
c. Research activities
d. Accounting
e. Gardening

Q.12.3 **The following items can be claimed by a non-dispensing doctor using F.P. 34D:**

a. Vaccines supplied free by the health authority
b. Pessaries
c. Ethyl chloride sprays
d. Contraceptive caps
e. Expired injections which have not been administered

Q.12.4 **Practice allowances and fees:**

a. In order to claim a temporary resident fee the patient must be staying in the practice area for 24 hours
b. Emergency treatment attracts a higher fee than a temporary resident claim
c. The F.P.C. will claim an emergency treatment fee back from the patient's registered doctor if he is in the same locality
d. Group practice allowance is paid to doctors who are in association and not in partnership
e. To qualify for supplementary practice allowance a principal must have at least 1000 patients on his list

For answers see over

Answers

A.12.1 a. F—This is an example of tertiary prevention as the disease is already established.
       b. T
       c. F—This is an example of primary prevention – preventing a disease from starting.
       d. F—Again, this is a primary preventive measure.
       e. T

A.12.2 a. T
       b. F
       c. F
       d. F
       e. F

A.12.3 a. F—But you can refuse health authority supplies and provide your own.
       b. T—They are classed as appliances.
       c. T—All local anaesthetics are claimable.
       d. T—But condoms are not!
       e. F

A.12.4 a. T—If the patient is staying for less than 24 hours, an immediate and necessary form should be completed.
       b. T
       c. T
       d. T
       e. T

Q.12.5 Cost rent scheme:

a. Only completely new premises are eligible for inclusion
b. There is no minimum cost for a project to be included
c. The practice can revert to notional rent at any time after completion of the project
d. A practice is not eligible for both improvement grants and inclusion in the cost rent scheme
e. The cost rent is only payable for 25 years

Q.12.6 Medical records:

a. An N.H.S. practitioner is legally obliged to keep records
b. The records held by a general practitioner are his legal property
c. The cost of conversion to A4 records is borne by the F.P.C.
d. An attached district nurse has legal right of access to the notes of a patient who has been referred to her by the G.P.
e. Patients have legal right of access to what a practitioner has extracted from his records for an insurance report

Q.12.7 The Joint Committee on Postgraduate Training for General Practice considers that a training practice must have:

a. A trainer who is a member of the R. C. G. P.
b. All continuation cards and letters in clinical record folders in date order
c. Patient summary cards
d. An age–sex register
e. Evidence of audit taking place within the practice

For answers see over

Answers

A.12.5 a. F—Substantial modification to existing premises is allowed.
        b. F—There was a minimum cost of £5070.00 in 1988.
        c. F—This can only be done every 3 years.
        d. F—But the amount awarded under the improvement grant is deducted from the final cost rent assessment.
        e. F—The cost rent can be paid as long as the premises are used for general practice services.

A.12.6 a. T
        b. F—They are the property of the Secretary of State.
        c. F—This is tax-allowable expense borne by the practice.
        d. F
        e. T—Recent legislation (1989) accords patients this right.

A.12.7 a. F
        b. T
        c. T
        d. T
        e. T

Q.12.8 Computer systems in general practice:

a. Patient information details can be downloaded from the F.P.C. computer at no charge to the practice
b. Once a system is installed, patients have immediate access to their records
c. Financial reimbursement for computer installation is available from the F.P.C.
d. Studies have shown that a computer terminal on a doctor's desk is acceptable to the majority of patients
e. The expense of installing a computer in a practitioner's home on which he organises the practice accounts is allowable against tax

Q.12.9 Cervical cytology claims:

a. A practitioner is allowed a fee for two smears done 1 month apart but one before the 35th birthday and one after it
b. A fee is claimable if the smear is performed by the practice nurse
c. A second fee is claimable if the smear was inadvertently destroyed by the laboratory
d. A second fee is claimable if the laboratory requests a retest because of abnormal cells
e. A fee is claimable for a patient of 22 years old who is gravida 3 para 0

Q.12.10 The practice nurse:

a. Legally the practice nurse must be a registered general nurse
b. Remuneration of 70% of her salary by the F.P.C. is independent of the number of other staff employed by the practice
c. Cervical smears done by a practice nurse do not qualify for an item of service fee
d. Immunisations done by the practice nurse do qualify for an item of service fee
e. Professional indemnity for the nurse is not required if she is employed by a general practitioner

For answers see over

Answers

A.12.8   a. F—The F.P.C. can charge.
            b. F—They have to make a written application and a charge can be made by the doctor.
            c. F—It is cheaper to employ people rather than computers.
            d. T
            e. T

A.12.9   a. T
            b. T
            c. T
            d. F
            e. T

A.12.10   a. F—An S. E. N. could be employed.
            b. F—A practice nurse is still part of the staffing allocation of two whole-time equivalents per doctor.
            c. F—They do if supervised by the doctor.
            d. T
            e. F—She should have her own indemnity or the practice can arrange it for her.

Q.12.11 The F.P.C. (Family Practitioner Committee)

a. is responsible for the services provided by dispensing chemists
b. is advised by the Local Medical Committee
c. is composed entirely of lay-members
d. is accountable to the Area Health Authority
e. receives its budget from the Area Health Authority

Q.12.12 Claims for immediate and necessary treatment:

a. A night visit fee can be claimed in addition if the visit is between 11.00 p.m. and 7.00 a.m.
b. A claim is payable if the patient has been seen as a temporary resident by another practice in the area within 14 days
c. The patient's signature is required
d. A claim is not payable if the patient is accepted within 3 months onto the practice list
e. The doctor must give any immediately necessary treatment for a period of 14 days once the form has been signed

Q.12.13 Patient participation groups

a. fail within 4 years in 25% of cases
b. are legally unable to raise funds for surgery equipment
c. have a national association
d. exist in the majority of practices within the United Kingdom
e. typically survive longer if there is doctor involvement

Q.12.14 National self-help groups exist for the following groups of patients:

a. Widows
b. Patients with psoriasis
c. Patients who have had a "cot death"
d. Osteo-arthritics
e. Families of alcoholics

For answers see over

Answers

A.12.11
a. T—And for those provided by general dental practitioners and ophthalmic medical practitioners as well as general practitioners.
b. T
c. F—Nominations are made by the L.M.C. for doctors to sit on the F.P.C.
d. F—It is accountable to the Secretary of State.
e. F—It receives direct funding from the D.H.S.S.

A.12.12
a. T
b. F
c. T—Unless he or she is too ill to sign.
d. T
e. T

A.12.13
a. T
b. F
c. T
d. F—Only about 100 practices have groups.
e. T

A.12.14
a. T—Cruse
b. T—Psoriasis Association.
c. T—Foundation for the Study of Infant Death.
d. T—Arthritis and Rheumatism Council.
e. T—Al-anon.

Q.12.15 **The General Medical Services Committee guidelines on practice booklets consider that the following information would be appropriate:**

a. Year of registration of the partners
b. Leisure and family interests of the partners
c. Any "special clinics" held within the practice
d. Appointments held outside the practice by the partners
e. Information about access for the disabled

Q.12.16 **Doctors' retainer scheme:**

a. It is only open to women doctors
b. A doctor participating in the scheme can work up to six sessions per week
c. The practice must select a suitable applicant
d. All practices are eligible to use the scheme
e. The employing practice is reimbursed by the F.P.C.

Q.12.17 **Night visit fees are paid in the following situations:**

a. A visit received at 06.55 hrs and attended at 07.15 hrs
b. A visit to a patient with an incomplete abortion at 02.00 hrs
c. A visit to a temporary resident received at 22.50 hrs and attended to at 23.30 hrs
d. A suturing at the surgery at 01.00 hrs
e. A home confinement at 06.00 hrs

Q.12.18 **Practitioners are allowed to receive:**

a. Financial gifts from their N.H.S. patients
b. Charges for private prescriptions
c. Charges for ear piercing
d. Charges for supplying information to a patient under the Data Protection Act
e. Reimbursement from a chemist after supplying him with samples obtained from a drug representative

For answers see over

Answers

A.12.15 a. T
              b. F
              c. T
              d. F
              e. T

A.12.16 a. F—Men can apply.
              b. F—He can work up to two sessions per week.
              c. F—The initiative must come from the participating doctor.
              d. F—Only suitable practices selected by the Regional Advisor
                   are eligible.
              e. T

A.12.17 a. F—It must be received and completed before 07.00 hrs.
              b. F—Fees are not payable for maternity cases.
              c. F—It must be received after 23.00 hrs.
              d. T
              e. F—See b.

A.12.18 a. F
              b. F
              c. T
              d. T
              e. F—This is illegal !!!

Q.12.19   Using an improvement grant from the F.P.C. a practice can

    a. extend the telephone system
    b. provide double glazing
    c. provide car parking facilities
    d. provide a sterilizer
    e. provide a new room for a trainee

Q.12.20   The following statements are true:

    a. The majority of practices operate personal list systems
    b. The majority of night visits are covered by deputising services
    c. There has been a decline in home visiting rates over the last decade
    d. The majority of doctors use an appointment system
    e. A practice receiving greater than 10% of its income from non-N.H.S. sources can lose reimbursement from the F.P.C.

For answers see over

Answers

A.12.19 a. T
           b. T
           c. T
           d. F—Equipment is not allowed.
           e. F

A.12.20 a. F—Only about 25% do so.
           b. F—Approximately 40% are.
           c. T—The figure is now about 0.5 visits per patient per year.
           d. T—Approximately 88% do so.
           e. T—It can lose rent and rates allowances and staff salary reimbursement.

13. Care of the Elderly

Q.13.1 Scurvy in the elderly:

a. Malaise and weakness are typical presenting symptoms
b. Associated gum changes are more common in edentulous patients
c. Anaemia is typically due to associated blood loss
d. Subperiosteal haemorrhages are more common than in children
e. Petechiae are characteristically found on the buttocks

Q.13.2 The following investigations have a raised upper normal value in the elderly:

a. ESR
b. Serum iron
c. White cell count
d. Serum cholestrol
e. Serum urea

Q.13.3 Osteoporosis in the elderly is associated with:

a. A history of back pain which remits spontaneously
b. A previous history of urinary stone
c. A raised serum phosphate
d. A dorsal kyphosis
e. An equal sex incidence

Q.13.4 Hypothermia in the elderly:

a. It is defined as an oral temperature of less than 35°C
b. More than 20% of patients have hypothyroidism
c. Heart block indicates a poor prognosis
d. Neck stiffness indicates meningism
e. Associated bronchopneumonia typically fails to show the usual physical signs

For answers see over

Answers

A.13.1 a. T
  b. F
  c. T
  d. F—The reverse is true; hence X-rays may be of little diagnostic value.
  e. F—They are characteristically found on posterior thighs, anterior forearms and abdomen.

A.13.2 a. T
  b. F
  c. F
  d. T
  e. T

A.13.3 a. T—Due to recurrent compression fractures.
  b. F
  c. F
  d. T
  e. F—It is commoner in females.

A.13.4 a. F—Oral temperatures are unreliable; a low reading rectal thermometer should be used and a temperature below 35°C on that is diagnostic.
  b. F—Only about 5% do so.
  c. F—It is found to some extent in most admissions.
  d. F—It is due to generalised muscle rigidity.
  e. T

Q.13.5 **The following exclude a diagnosis of hyperthyroidism in the elderly:**

    a. Constipation
    b. Absence of tachycardia
    c. Reduced appetite
    d. Apathy
    e. Obesity

Q.13.6 **The following factors affect drug metabolism in the elderly:**

    a. Decreased absorption from the gut
    b. Decreased muscle mass
    c. Decreased renal excretion
    d. Decreased cardiac output
    e. Decreased hepatic blood flow

Q.13.7 **Insomnia in the elderly:**

    a. The total time sleeping is less than in those younger
    b. Early waking in the absence of other symptoms indicates depression
    c. Beta-blockers are more likely to produce nightmares in the elderly patient
    d. Frequent waking indicates disturbed mood
    e. Chlormethiazole has a short duration of action

Q.13.8 **Breast cancer in the elderly:**

    a. Elderly patients are less likely to report a breast lump than younger patients
    b. Pain in the breast is a typical presenting feature in the elderly
    c. The incidence of breast cancer decreases after the age of 65
    d. Less women over 65 die of breast cancer than women under 65 years of age
    e. Tamoxifen is contra-indicated in the over 75 year old

For answers see over

Answers

A.13.5 a. F—Constipation is more common than diarrhoea in the elderly thyrotoxic.
        b. F—25% have no tachycardia at diagnosis.
        c. F
        d. F
        e. F

A.13.6 a. F—As most absorption occurs by passive diffusion.
        b. T
        c. T—Due to decreased renal tubular function.
        d. T
        e. T—Hepatic blood flow almost halves between 30 and 75 years of age.

A.13.7 a. T
        b. F—Early waking is usual.
        c. T
        d. F—Up to six times at least is normal.
        e. T

A.13.8 a. T—They delay reporting on average for 3 months.
        b. F—Breast cancer is typically painless in all age groups.
        c. F—It increases.
        d. F
        e. F

Q.13.9   Hearing loss in the elderly:

    a. It is typically in the lower frequencies
    b. Presbyacusis typically starts in the 70s
    c. Hearing aids under the N.H.S. are charged for
    d. Hearing aids typically make tinnitus worse
    e. Body-worn hearing aids are inappropriate in the elderly

Q.13.10   Urinary incontinence in old age:

    a. A carefully timed toilet regime is typically of benefit
    b. Hypnotics typically reduce nocturnal incontinence
    c. If it is treated with a catheter, bacilluria is an indication for antibiotic therapy
    d. Constipation has been shown to be a precipitating factor
    e. An association with atropic vaginitis has been shown

For answers see over

Answers

A.13.9   a. F—Hearing in the lower frequencies is usually well preserved.
            b. F—It often starts in the 50 year old.
            c. F—They are issued free to the elderly at present.
            d. F—They often mask it.
            e. F—Their operation is often easier.

A.13.10   a. T
            b. F—Typically it would be increased.
            c. F—Only if symptomatic.
            d. T
            e. T—Sphincter efficiency is compromised in such cases.

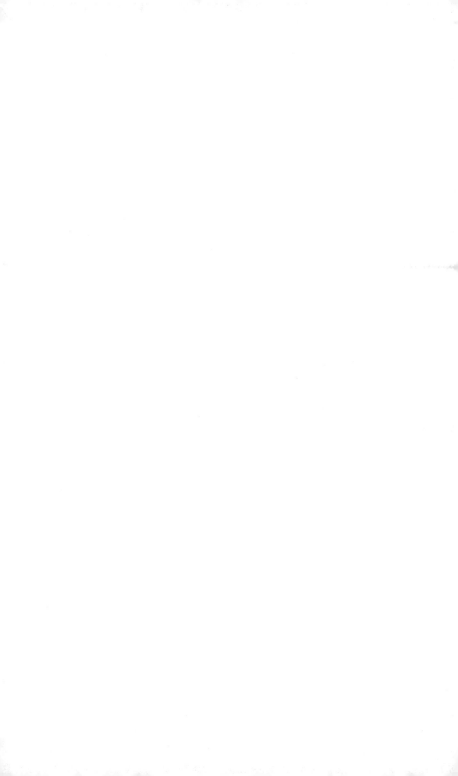

14. *Physical Medicine/Trauma*

Q.14.1 Reactive arthritis

a. occurs secondary to bacterial diarrhoea
b. typically occurs in the 16–30 year age group
c. has a poor prognosis if symptoms persist after 3 months
d. is associated with the HLA-B27 antibody
e. typically affects the joints of the upper limbs

Q.14.2 Arthritis has been shown to be associated with the following infections:

a. Measles
b. Mumps
c. Mycoplasma pneumonia
d. Viral hepatitis A
e. *Campylobacter*

Q.14.3 Acute traumatic arthritis:

a. The ESR is typically raised
b. Joint aspiration has been shown to be the treatment of choice
c. Intra-articular steroids, if given in the acute stage, have been shown to be free of risk
d. Spontaneous recovery occurs within 6 weeks in the majority of cases
e. Osteo-arthritis is a typical sequel to a single episode which resolves spontaneously

Q.14.4 Rheumatoid arthritis:

a. It is commoner in females
b. In the majority of cases it commences with an acute arthritis
c. A positive antinuclear factor would indicate an incorrect diagnosis
d. Erosions are typical early X-ray changes
e. Anaemia is typically independent of disease activity

For answers see over

Answers

A.14.1   a. T—Including shigella, salmonella and campylobacter.
          b. T—With males being more affected than females.
          c. F—Symptoms may last for more than 6 months with complete recovery.
          d. T—10% of the population has this antibody.
          e. F—The upper limbs are rarely affected; the condition typically affects the ankles, knees and toe joints.

A.14.2   a. F
          b. T—Arthritis occurs in 0.5% of infections approximately 3–4 weeks after the parotitis and usually affecting the knees and ankles.
          c. T—Arthritis is a rare complication; it responds to antibiotic treatment.
          d. T—Arthritis is commoner in viral hepatitis B but it does occur in type A; the proximal interphalangeal joints of the hands are commonly affected; involvement is usually symmetrical.
          e. T—Reactive arthritis may occur 5–14 days after the preceding gut infection.

A.14.3   a. F—This would indicate another cause for the problem.
          b. F—It is potentially hazardous, but may speed recovery if the effusion is a large tense haemarthrosis.
          c. F—They are best avoided, especially in sportsmen with recurrent injury; usually one injection is recommended in a case that is failing to respond to other measures.
          d. T—Hence the need for conservative measures of rest and physiotherapy with adequate anti-inflammatory analgesics.
          e. F—Osteo-arthritis usually only occurs if the trauma is repeated or there is associated bony injury.

A.14.4   a. T—This is a basic fact! The female–male ratio is 3:1.
          b. F—Only 15% of cases commence acutely; the commonest presentation is an insidious onset.
          c. F—It is common in rheumatoid arthritis, but a positive anti-DNA antibody test never occurs and would indicate SLE.
          d. T—Especially in the hands and feet.
          e. F—Anaemia is common and parallels activity of the disease.

Q.14.5 Arthritis following an infection with rubella

a. is monarticular in the majority of cases
b. is commoner in females
c. is typically synchronous with the rash
d. has been shown to occur after rubella vaccination
e. typically resolves completely

Q.14.6 Polymyalgia rheumatica:

a. It is the commonest inflammatory rheumatic disease in the elderly
b. It characteristically causes severe stiffness late in the day
c. Anorexia and weight loss are typical presenting features
d. The initial ESR result is a guide to severity and prognosis
e. NSAIDs are the treatment of choice whilst awaiting the results of further investigations

Q.14.7 Carpel tunnel syndrome:

a. Presentation is typically unilateral
b. Symptoms are characteristically worse at night
c. NSAIDs are the treatment of choice
d. Pain radiating to the shoulder suggests that the diagnosis is incorrect
e. Forced flexion of the wrist typically will reproduce the symptoms

Q.14.8 Oral gold therapy in rheumatoid arthritis

a. is cheaper than injectable treatment in equivalent dosage
b. does not require regular urine testing for protein
c. has been shown to be more effective than placebo
d. has been shown to more effective than injectable treatment
e. more commonly causes diarrhoea than does injectable treatment

For answers see over

Answers

A.14.5 a. F—It is usually bilateral and symmetrical, affecting meta-carpophalangeal and proximal interphalangeal joints.
        b. F—The sex incidence is equal.
        c. T—It may start a few days before or after the rash.
        d. T—Usually 2–4 weeks after the injection.
        e. T

A.14.6 a. T—It has an incidence of 1.5%.
        b. F—Early morning stiffness is characteristic.
        c. T—It is often accompanied by general malaise.
        d. F
        e. F—Steroids should be started as soon as possible.

A.14.7 a. F—It is usually bilateral but worse on the dominant side.
        b. T
        c. F—They increase fluid retention and may make symptoms worse.
        d. F—Pain can radiate both up and down the median nerve.
        e. T—As will a tight band around the wrist or forearm.

A.14.8 a. F—It is almost twice the price.
        b. F—Proteinuria occurs in 4% of patients and urine should be tested monthly.
        c. T
        d. F
        e. T—40% vs 18%.

Q.14.9   Gout:

    a. A raised serum uric acid level establishes the diagnosis
    b. Urate-lowering drugs should be started during the acute attack
    c. Radiological changes occur early in the disease
    d. The majority of cases occur in women
    e. There is typically a strong family history

Q.14.10   A diagnosis of prolapsed intervertebral disc would be supported by:

    a. Pain which is worse on resting
    b. Pain which is unremitting in character
    c. Bilateral symmetrical nerve involvement
    d. Compressions of a single nerve root
    e. No evidence of nerve compression

Q.14.11   Septic arthritis:

    a. There is typically an associated anaemia
    b. The ESR is characteristically raised
    c. Radiology of the affected joint in the first 48 hours will produce a characteristic appearance
    d. Rigors are a typical presenting feature
    e. The commonest infecting organism is *Haemophilus influenzae*

Q.14.12   Rheumatoid nodules

    a. are associated with an adverse prognosis
    b. are characteristically associated with seropostivity
    c. are found in less than 5% of patients with rheumatoid arthritis
    d. occur only in subcutaneous tissues
    e. typically occur over bony prominences

For answers see over

Answers

A.14.9 a. F—Diagnosis requires identification of uric acid crystals in the synovial fluid.
b. F—They should never be given acutely.
c. F—They usually occur in the late stages when the diagnosis is well established.
d. F—It is much more common in males.
e. T—A hereditary defect of purine metabolism is typical.

A.14.10 a. F—This indicates another cause such as infection, tumour or metabolic disease.
b. F—Again, this indicates another cause.
c. F
d. T—If more than one root is involved the diagnosis is less likely.
e. F

A.14.11 a. F—Even the white cell count may be normal in the early stages.
b. T
c. F—Radiology is unhelpful in the early stages.
d. T
e. F—This is only true at less than 2 years of age; after that *Staphylococcus aureus* is more common.

A.14.12 a. T
b. T
c. F—They are found in approximately 20%–30% of cases.
d. F—They can occur in lung, pleura, myocardium, pericardium and tendon sheaths.
e. T—Classic sites are the forearm and elbow.

Q.14.13 Ankylosing spondylitis

a. has been shown to be associated with erythema nodosum
b. characteristically involves back pain which is worse when waking
c. is a cause of renal failure
d. is associated with aortic incompetence
e. is associated with conjuctivitis

Q.14.14 Rheumatoid arthritis and pregnancy:

a. The incidence of abortion is increased
b. The majority of patients undergo remission during pregnancy
c. Post-partum deterioration occurs in the majority of patients
d. Obstetric complications have been shown to be increased
e. Continuing lactation prevents post-partum relapse

Q.14.15 Paget's disease of the bone

a. typically involves elevation of serum alkaline phosphatase
b. typically involves nocturnal bone pain
c. is associated with the development of osteosarcoma
d. is commoner in men than women
e. has been shown to cause pathological fractures

For answers see over

Answers

A.14.13   a. F
        b. T
        c. T—Due to secondary amyloidosis.
        d. T—In 4% there is a non-specific aortitis.
        e. F—It is usually associated with iritis.

A.14.14   a. F
        b. T—75% undergo remission.
        c. T—It usually does so in the second month after delivery.
        d. F
        e. F—Deterioration is independent of breast-feeding.

A.14.15   a. T
        b. T
        c. T—Osteosarcoma develops in approximately 1% of cases and is usually highly malignant.
        d. F—The incidence is equal in males and females.
        e. T

15. *Infectious Disease*

Q.15.1   Sterilisation:

a. Micro-organisms are more resistant to dry heat than to moist heat
b. Boiling at 100°C kills spores
c. Chlorhexidine is inactivated by soap
d. Hexachlorophene has been shown to be neurotoxic
e. Immersion in 75% alcohol kills spores

Q.15.2   Enteritis caused by rotavirus

a. is commoner in the warmer months of the year
b. has an incubation period of 1 week
c. is associated with upper respiratory symptoms
d. typically causes an asymptomatic infection in neonates
e. has a peak incidence in the 6–24 month age group

Q.15.3   MMR (mumps, measles and rubella) vaccine:

a. It is contra-indicated if measles vaccine has been given previously
b. It should be given to asymptomatic HIV-positive children
c. Booster injections should be given between 10 and 14 years of age
d. Immunoglobulin can be given concurrently
e. Epilepsy in a first-degree relative is an absolute contra-indication

Q.15.4   Recurrent genital herpes infection

a. is significantly helped by topical acyclovir
b. tends to diminish over time
c. is due to herpes simplex virus I in the majority of cases
d. is precipitated by menstruation
e. is not transmitted once the lesions are painless

For answers see over

Answers

A.15.1 a. T—Dry heat penetrates slowly; therefore longer exposure times and greater temperatures are needed.
        b. F—It only kills vegetative organisms, not spores.
        c. T
        d. T
        e. F—It is bactericidal to vegetative organisms only.

A.15.2 a. F—It is commoner in the winter months.
        b. F—The incubation period is 1–2 days.
        c. T—Cough, nasal discharge and otitis media are associated.
        d. T—It usually causes an asymptomatic infection in adults and in neonates (who have maternal antibodies).
        e. T—This is so-called weanling diarrhoea; 90% of 2 year olds have antibodies.

A.15.3 a. F
        b. T—Use in symptomatic children is still controversial.
        c. F—It is a single dose vaccine.
        d. F—It inactivates the vaccine.
        e. F

A.15.4 a. F—It is helped by oral acyclovir but only while the drug is being taken
        b. T
        c. F—It is due to type II virus in 90% of cases.
        d. T—And by intercourse.
        e. F—It can be transmitted to a sexual partner up to 2 weeks after the pain has disappeared.

Q.15.5 Mycoplasma (atypical) pneumonia

   a. has a peak incidence in young adults
   b. typically causes pleuritic symptoms
   c. has an insidious onset.
   d. is best treated by a synthetic penicillin
   e. has been shown to have neurological complications

Q.15.6 Chickenpox:

   a. If present before the 20th week of pregnancy it is harmless to the foetus
   b. The course in adults is typically less complicated
   c. It has been shown to cause Reye's syndrome
   d. It is potentially fatal in immune-deficient children
   e. Varicella virus vaccine is available

Q.15.7 Enteroviruses have been shown to cause:

   a. Hepatitis A
   b. Hand, foot and mouth disease
   c. Epidemic myalgia
   d. Aseptic meningitis
   e. Endocarditis

Q.15.8 Gonococcal arthritis:

   a. Men are more commonly affected.
   b. It typically presents 1 month after the original infection
   c. A high ESR is characteristic
   d. The knee is the commonest joint involved
   e. Effective antibiotic treatment produces complete resolution within 1 month

For answers see over

Answers

A.15.5 a. F—The peak incidence is in the 5–15 age group.
        b. F—Pleurisy is a rare problem.
        c. T—Usually with cough, malaise and fever.
        d. F—It is resistant to them; it is best treated with tetracyclines or erythromycin.
        e. T—In 6%–7% of cases it causes a variety of complications, including meningitis, polyneuritis and cranial nerve palsy.

A.15.6 a. F—It can lead to cerebral atrophy and optic atrophy and is usually considered grounds for termination.
        b. F—Complications are much commoner in adults.
        c. T
        d. T—It needs vigorous treatment with antiviral agents.
        e. T—It is recommended that it be given to children with leukaemia before they are immunosuppressed.

A.15.7 a. T—Enterovirus 72.
        b. T—Coxsackie A16.
        c. T—Coxsackie B6.
        d. T—Polio virus and other echo and Coxsackie viruses.
        e. T—Coxsackie B group.

A.15.8 a. F—It is four times commoner in females.
        b. F—It presents 3–17 days later, usually after 14 days.
        c. F—If raised, the ESR is only slightly above normal.
        d. T—The knee involved in 75% of cases.
        e. T

Q.15.9 **The following organisms have been shown to occur in the flora of a normal pharynx:**

    a. *Streptococcus pneumoniae*
    b. *Haemophilus influenzae*
    c. Alpha haemolytic streptococci
    d. *Candida* species
    e. Diptheroids

Q.15.10 **Head lice**

    a. are typically found on the vertex of the scalp
    b. live for 3 months or more
    c. are treated with malathion applied to wet hair
    d. are able to hop or jump from one head to another host
    e. can be carried by family pets

For answers see over

Answers

A.15.9 a. T—It occurs in most adults and children.
          b. T— Again, it is found in most adults and children.
          c. T—It is the dominant aerobic species.
          d. T
          e. T

A.15.10 a. F—They are usually found behind the ears and on the back of the neck.
          b. F—They only live for 1 month.
          c. F—It should be applied to dry hair and allowed to dry without the aid of a hair dryer.
          d. F—They can be transferred only by direct contact; they are also unable to fly.
          e. F

Suggested Reading

Apart from the usual magazines that arrive with monotonous regularity on your desk, I would advise a look at some of the following:

General Medicine

Cormack J, Marinker M, Morrell D (1987) Practice, a handbook of primary medical care. Kluwer Medical, London
Hodgkin K (1985) Towards earlier diagnosis (1985). Churchill Livingstone, Edinburgh
Davies IJT (1985) Postgraduate medicine. Lloyd Luke, London

Psychiatry

Tredgold R, Wolff H (1975) U.C.H. handbook of psychiatry. Duckworth
Turner RM, Williams P (1986) Psychological disorders. MTP, Lancaster

Obstetrics and Gynaecology

McPherson A, Anderson A (1987) Women's problems in general practice. Oxford University Press, Oxford
Kaye P (1986) Notes for the D. R. C. O. G. Churchill Livingstone, Edinburgh
Marsh GN (1987) Modern obstetrics in general practice. Oxford University Press, Oxford

Therapeutics

British National Formulary (1989)
Brodie MJ, Harrison I (1986) Practical prescribing. Churchill Livingstone, Edinburgh

Paediatrics

Modell M, Boyd R (1984) Paediatric problems in general practice. Oxford University Press, Oxford
Valman HB (1984) The first year of life. B. M. J.
Valman HB (1988) ABC of one to seven. B. M. J.

ENT

Ludman H (1988) ABC of ear, nose and throat. B. M. J.
Wright T (1988) Dizziness. Croom Helm, London

Dermatology

Buxton PK (1988) ABC of dermatology. B. M. J.
McKie R (1986) Clinical dermatology. Oxford University Press, Oxford

Ophthalmology

Gardiner PA (1979) ABC of ophthalmology. B. M. J.
Jackson CRS, Finlay RD (1986) The eye in general practice. Churchill Livingstone, Edinburgh

Legal and Ethical

Knight B (1987) Legal aspects of medical practice. Churchill Livingstone, Edinburgh

Epidemiology and Research

Howie J (1979) Research in general practice. Croom Helm, London
Castle WM (1977) Statistics in small doses. Churchill Livingstone, Edinburgh
Fry J (1984) Common diseases. MTP, Lancaster

Practice Organisation

Jones RVH, Bolden RJ, Pereira Gray DJ, Hall MS (1988) Running a practice. Croom Helm, London
Pritchard PMM (1985) Management in general practice. Oxford University Press, Oxford

Care of the Elderly

Wright WB (1986) The elderly patient. Springer, Berlin Heidelberg New York
Wilcock GK, Gray JAM, Pritchard PMM (1983) Geriatric problems in general practice. Oxford University Press, Oxford

Physical Medicine

Huskisson EC, Dudley Hart F (1978) Joint disease. John Wright, Bristol
Newell RLM Turner JG (1985) Orthopaedic disorders in general practice. Butterworths, London

Infectious Disease

Benn RAV (1985) Aids to microbiology and infectious disease. Churchill Livingstone, Edinburgh